Clinics in Developmental Medicine No. 167
PRECHTL'S METHOD ON THE QUALITATIVE
ASSESSMENT OF GENERAL MOVEMENTS IN
PRETERM, TERM AND YOUNG INFANTS

© 2004 Mac Keith Press
2nd Floor, Rankin Building, 139-143 Bermondsey Street, London se1 3uw

Editor: Hilary M. Hart
Managing Editor: Michael Pountney
Project Manager: Sarah Pearsall

First published in this edition 2004
Reprinted 2012, 2015, 2016, 2017, 2019, 2022, 2023

British Library Cataloguing-in-Publication data
A catalogue record for this book is available from the British Library

ISSN (hardback): 978-1-898683-40-7
ISBN (paperback): 978-1-898683-62-9

Typeset by Keystroke, Jacaranda Lodge, Wolverhampton
Printed by Hobbs the Printers Ltd, Totton, Hampshire

Clinics in Developmental Medicine No. 167

Prechtl's Method on the Qualitative Assessment of General Movements in Preterm, Term and Young Infants

CHRISTA EINSPIELER
Medical University of Graz, Austria

HEINZ F.R. PRECHTL
University of Groningen, the Netherlands and
Medical University of Graz, Austria

AREND F. BOS
University of Groningen, the Netherlands

FABRIZIO FERRARI
University of Modena and Reggio Emilia, Italy

GIOVANNI CIONI
University of Pisa and Stella Maris Foundation, Italy

2004
Mac Keith Press

Il moto é causa d'ogni vita.

LEONARDO DA VINCI

Ein Kind, sich bewegend, erzählt mit Berührung sein Leben der Zeit.

GRAZ 2003

CONTENTS

AUTHORS' APPOINTMENTS

Christa Einspieler   Professor of Physiology, Medical University of Graz, Austria

Heinz F.R. Prechtl   Professor Emeritus of Developmental Neurology, University of Groningen, the Netherlands and Honorary Professor, Medical University of Graz, Austria

Arend F. Bos   Professor of Neonatology, University of Groningen, the Netherlands

Fabrizio Ferrari   Professor of Paediatrics, University of Modena and Reggio Emilia, Italy

Giovanni Cioni   Professor of Child Neurology and Psychiatry, University of Pisa and Stella Maris Foundation, Italy

ACKNOWLEDGEMENTS

Christa Einspieler would like to express her sincere gratitude to her cousin Dr Uli Todoroff for creating a unique atmosphere in a medieval stone house in Vinci, Tuscany. This book could not have been written without her continuous supply of cooled water, fresh salads, and dried apricots, and her battle against aggressive mosquitoes during three hot summer weeks in 2003.

INTRODUCTION: HOW IT ALL CAME ABOUT

Heinz F.R. Prechtl

The key to understanding and fully appreciating a newly introduced assessment technique is to trace its history. One question frequently raised during the training courses on GM assessment is: 'How did you hit on the idea of a qualitative assessment of general movements as a specific predictor for neurological impairment?' Below I will outline the historical background of the 'whys' and 'wherefores' that finally led to the rationale for this new method.

As is invariably the case with the answer to a seemingly simple question, the approach that led to the final solution was far from direct. Indeed, I have travelled down a long and winding path to reach the final goal. From my initial attempts to design a reliable and standardised method for a neurological examination of the fullterm neonate in the late 1950s and early 1960s, my interest was focused on the early assessment of brain dysfunction (Prechtl and Beintema 1964, Prechtl 1977). At the time, adult neurologists considered such a neurological technique illusory because of the inconsistencies of reflex and response patterns in newborn infants. What was as yet unknown was the high dependency of these patterns on the infant's behavioural state. As soon as this problem was solved (see Prechtl 1974), normal infants did respond consistently to the eliciting stimuli. So now, if they did not respond despite being in the right behavioural state, it meant that something must be wrong and it was then an abnormal neurological sign.

Classic neurological assessment has two shortcomings, although it is still an indispensable tool even today. The first problem is twofold: a shortened version is unreliable and to carry out a reliable (and therefore detailed and longer) version is perceived as too time-consuming. However, it should be remembered that the nervous system is the most complex and complicated organ of any organism. This aspect is all too often not appreciated sufficiently. The second shortcoming is that the classic neurological examination can reveal the acute condition of the infant's nervous system but it lacks the power to make a specific prognosis of neurological outcome. From detailed follow-up studies and group comparisons we knew the chance rate of normal outcome, minor abnormalities and severe impairment. At the level of the individual infant and its parents, this approach was rather much of a gamble and more of a burden than a help. Hence, there was felt to be a great need for a technique of early neurological assessment that was at once cost-effective, easy to learn, quick, and had a high individual predictive power.

The path that led to the method that met these requirements was long and rather complicated as it first carried us to completely unrelated problems. In the 1970s, after already having worked for some 25 years in the field of infant neurology, I started wondering about the prenatal development of the many spontaneous motor patterns seen in the newborn. Birth could not be the starting point; these motor patterns must have a longer, prenatal history. Because, until then, only reflex studies had been carried out on aborted foetuses (Minkowski 1928, Hooker 1952), the advent of advanced real time ultrasound heralded the beginning of non-invasive, intra-uterine observation of the foetus. It would enable us to study the undisturbed foetus in its natural environment. However, at the time, ultrasound equipment had not yet improved sufficiently to allow the observation of foetal movements. I decided to carry out a preparatory study with the unaided eye of unstimulated preterm infants, just to observe what they do if left alone, and perhaps to enable me later to recognise certain movement patterns in the foetus (Prechtl et al 1979). This was an unusual approach then and unfortunately it still is.

A group of very low-risk preterm infants was painstakingly selected. These infants showed a large variety of spontaneous movement patterns, which could be easily recognised each time they occurred. It was amazing how many specific motor patterns were endogenously generated without any external stimulation (Prechtl et al 1979). These observations contrasted dramatically with the concept of a passive nervous system but for the grace of many sensory inputs. Our observations were an eye-opener and, armed with this knowledge, the foetal studies could commence in 1981 – with technically more advanced ultrasound equipment (de Vries JIP et al 1982, 1984, 1985, 1987, 1988). Again, our focus of interest was the complex repertoire of spontaneous movements and our findings confirmed that postnatal behaviour has indeed a long prenatal history. But, there was another important discovery: the continuity from prenatal to postnatal life of many neural functions (Prechtl 1984a). Only at 3 months does the nervous system become adapted to the requirements of extra-uterine life. Of course, this holds true for non-vital functions only (Prechtl 1984b, 1986).

All of this would not have given a clue to a new assessment technique had we not also collected similar observations on high-risk preterm infants. Our original expectation of a significant difference in the incidence of the various specific movement patterns between the low-risk and the high-risk infants was not confirmed (Prechtl and Nolte 1984). However, we suspected that the high-risk infant moves differently from the normal infant. This marked the beginning of a new approach to assessing the young nervous system, even if it was not yet sufficiently specified. Significant help came from newly developed video-recording equipment. In contrast to previously used cine-filming, video allowed us to view the recording immediately after the session, and we could even replay it at different speeds.

Another crucial technical development was the method of ultrasound brain examination. We combined both techniques – the new video technology and brain ultrasound – and replicated the previous observational studies on a selection of cases with or without brain ultrasound abnormalities and video-recorded their spontaneous movement patterns (Ferrari et al 1990, Prechtl 1990). The main focus was on the so-called general movements which had first been described in the observational study of normal preterm infants (Prechtl et al 1979). The study by Ferrari et al (1990) on preterm and term infants was the convincing first indication that we were on the right path: the qualitative assessment of general movements, those most frequently occurring, long-lasting and complex spontaneous movement patterns, is what really counts and not the quantitative differences.

The problem that now confronted us was that if you cannot count and reproduce the differences in numbers, might the technique not be too subjective? Therefore, a crucial importance for our new technique was the interscorer agreement, as the qualitative assessment of general movements is based on visual Gestalt perception. Indeed, an interscorer agreement of 90 per cent is sufficiently high (see Chapter 5). It should be realised that visual Gestalt perception is an excellent scientific tool. The importance of visual observation in daily clinical routine and research was recently emphasised by Bax (2002) in his editorial 'Clinical assessment still matters'.

The attention shift from exclusively reflex to spontaneous movements in the early neurological assessment again has a historical background. The change of paradigm from a passive to an active and endogenously generating central nervous system must have consequences for neurological assessment. I must admit that the realisation of the importance of spontaneous motor activity, and of general movements in particular, came after our empirical findings.

Classic neurophysiologists studied neural functions on the basis of experimentally impaired neural systems. The quantitative relationship between the sensory input and the reflex (motor) output was the focus of their attention (Sherrington 1906). Clear-cut, quantitative results could only be obtained by excluding the nuisance of the interfering spontaneous activity. This led to historical distortions of the concept of neural functions, distortions that have not yet been fully overcome to this day. Neurology has come a long way to rediscover the importance of endogenously generated activity, particularly in the young organism, and to place reflex activity there where it is of biological significance.

I would like to conclude by saying: if reflexes are performed more consistently by de-cerebrated animals, reflexes cannot be the best way to study the consequences of brain impairment. On the other hand, the qualitative assessment of spontaneous activity is a sensitive indicator of certain neurological impairments and, hence, opens up a window into the brain.

This then is the rationale for the method described in this book and the way it came about.

Videos: Videos to accompany 15 cases selected from the book are FREE with every book purchased through the Mac Keith Press website. Each is of about one minute in duration and demonstrates the different age-specific movement patterns.

Contact admin@mackeith.co.uk for free access if you have purchased the book from another bookseller.

1
BASIC CONCEPTS OF DEVELOPMENTAL NEUROLOGY

**The assessment of general movements within the concept
of ontogenetic adaptation**

During the past 40 years, research in developmental neurology has provided a number of significant new paradigms on the functional development of the human nervous system. One of the most fundamental new insights is the concept of ontogenetic adaptation with its far-reaching consequences (Oppenheim 1984). This concept acknowledges that during the development of the individual the functional repertoire of the developing neural structure must meet the requirements of the organism and its environment (Prechtl 2001a).

However, in comparison to neonatal infra-human primates the human neonate is less adapted to the extra-uterine environment as far as non-vital functions are concerned. The human pregnancy is relatively short in respect to the allometric measurements of maternal body weight, brain weight, metabolic rate and maximal life span (Prechtl 1986, 2001a). The first two months after term are in a certain way a continuation of foetal behaviour. At the third month a major transformation of many neural functions occurs, and only then is the young human infant much more adapted to the requirements of extra-uterine life (Prechtl 1984a, 1984b). Such a delay seems specific for the human species (Prechtl 2001a).

At 3 months the infant's muscle power increases; the body posture changes from a body-oriented to a space-oriented postural control (Prechtl 1989a); the sucking pattern changes from tongue peristaltic movements to a new pattern of sucking with open corners of the mouth (Iwayama and Eishima 1997); control of visual attention and binocular vision develop (Braddick and Atkinson 1983, Atkinson 1984a, 1984b); social smiling and pleasure vocalisation while looking towards the caregiver occur (van Wulfften Palthe and Hopkins 1984); and general movements change their form (Hopkins and Prechtl 1984, Prechtl 1986, 2001a). This list is far from complete. These changes occur during a relatively short period of a few weeks. The increased strength of the muscles makes movements more effective; the switch-on of antigravity postures and orientation of the infant in space, as well as the onset of true social interaction with the caregiver, are signs of a more effective ontogenetic adaptation to the new environment. It must be assumed that this obvious developmental delay in the human species can be compensated by the effectiveness of the larger brain with higher 'intelligence' of caregiving in the parents (Prechtl 1984b, 1986).

With the exception of the above-mentioned delay, the developing organism is during each developmental stage adapted to the internal and external requirements. Therefore, each developmental stage must be studied in its own right and not in relation to later developmental stages. At different ages we are dealing with qualitatively different nervous systems. These differences comprise the structure as well as the functional repertoire. A consequence of the age-specific difference of the developing nervous system is the age-specific vulnerability of the nervous tissue. Hence, the clinical consequence is that age-specific signs and syndromes require age-adequate diagnostic procedures (Prechtl 2001a). Of course, any neurological examination and assessment must meet this requirement. Prechtl's method of qualitative assessment of general movements takes full account of the age-specificity and the ontogenetic adaptation (Fig. 1.1).

From reflex and tonus testing to observation of spontaneous movements
If we consider the work of classic neurophysiology, which is associated with the name of the eminent Sir Charles Sherrington, it becomes clear that de-cerebrated animals and spinal preparations formed the basis of detailed studies on reflexes and responses to all kinds of sensory stimulation. With this ingenious trick it was possible to get rid of the annoying interference stemming from the spontaneous activity of the nervous system (Sherrington 1906). Only under de-cerebration did it become possible to study in detail a stable, quantitative relationship between sensory input and reflexive motor output. Having accepted this fact, we should not be too surprised if, in general, reflexes are poor indicators of brain function and dysfunction.

On the other hand, as a logical consequence of all the experiments in the realm of classic neurophysiology, spontaneous motility, as the expression of spontaneous neural activity, cannot but be an excellent marker of brain lesions. Nevertheless, it may still be surprising that this fact has been overlooked for such a long time. The enormous success of

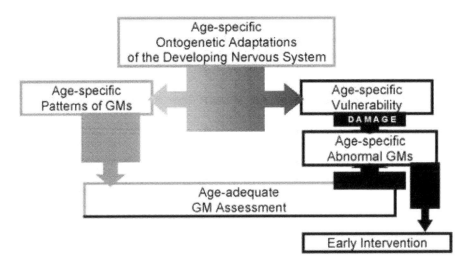

Fig. 1.1 General movement assessment as a method of developmental neurology with its basic concept of ontogenetic adaptation and its consequences.

the classic stimulus–response investigations has created a tremendous bias in our thinking about the function of the nervous system (Prechtl 1997a, 2001a). Hence, it took a long time to change paradigms. In part, this task was left to the young field of developmental neurology during the second half of the twentieth century.

The concept of tonus or tone was introduced into the neurology of the young infant by the eminent adult neurologist Andre-Thomas. His outstanding book on cerebellar diseases dealt with tonus changes as an important clinical sign. His later co-operation with S. Saint-Anne Dargassies brought his ideas of tonus testing to infant neurology (Thomas and Saint-Anne Dargassies 1952). This tradition continued with Claudine Amiel-Tison (Amiel-Tison and Grenier 1983) and the Dubowitzs (Dubowitz and Dubowitz 1981, Dubowitz et al 1999). Regrettably, the definition and assessment of tonus are not standardised and vary greatly. Clinical experience indicates the inconsistent character of tonus in young infants, and the inter-observer agreement is weak. Severe cases of hypotonia and hypertonia are exceptions to the case in point and are clinically important. However, during the first weeks of life hypotonia and hypertonia are not specific signs of later neurological deficits (Prechtl 1997a, 2001a).

In the observation of infants the interest has changed from the analysis of the capacities to respond to a manifold of sensory stimulations, to the observation of the un-stimulated infant. Naturalistic observations led to the conclusion of the dominance of spontaneous behaviour, i.e. behaviour not generated by sensory stimulation.

Two investigations must be mentioned. The pioneer work by Arnold Gesell (1945) was based on a developmental concept, which was interpreted as a genetically determined maturation of neural functions. His interest was focused on a developmental test, which would enable the examiner to discriminate between normal milestones and retarded development. The description of the various motor patterns at different ages was based on cine-film of the infants and children. However, the database was relatively small, and therefore the Zurich study (Largo et al 1990, Largo 1993) made improvements and corrections to the Gesell study.

The other work along similar lines was carried out by the psychologist Myrtle McGraw (1943). In a period dominated by behaviourism it was understandable that the word 'spontaneous' was in quotation marks. McGraw said about the neonate: 'Perhaps the most striking aspect of newborn behaviour is general motility. The so-called "spontaneous" behaviour of the neonate has attracted the attention of many investigators. It is the incoordination and lack of form which differentiates spontaneous movements from other (reflexive) neuromuscular activity' (1943: 18-19).

This view has changed dramatically since unstimulated foetuses, preterm and term infants have been systematically and longitudinally observed (Prechtl et al 1979, Cioni et al 1989, Prechtl 1989b, Cioni and Prechtl 1990). In fact, all foetal movement patterns, which are endogenously generated by the unstimulated nervous system, are distinctly patterned right from the first onset at about 8 to 9 weeks postmenstrual age. There exists no phase of uncoordinated and amorphic movements (Prechtl 1989b, 2001b). A rich repertoire develops within a few weeks, which continues after birth unchanged for the first two to three months (Prechtl 1992).

The question of how spontaneous movements are generated by the nervous system has recently been answered. Results from developmental neurobiology are rapidly accumulating convincing evidence that, under normal conditions, the young nervous system is to a large extent an active organ (see Chapter 2). The spontaneous motility of foetuses, preterm and term infants as well as infants during their first months of life has great clinical significance (e.g. Ferrari et al 1990, Prechtl and Einspieler 1997, Prechtl et al 1997b). It proves to be an important functional indicator of brain dysfunction at a very early age and tells us more about the young nervous system than any amount of reflex testing does (Prechtl 1997a, 2001a).

2
WHAT ARE SPONTANEOUS MOVEMENTS?

That the young human nervous system endogenously, i.e. without being constantly triggered by specific sensory input, generates a variety of motor patterns has been known for more than a century. William Preyer (1885) was fully aware of this fact, but it was forgotten for a while, only to be rediscovered later in animals by Erich von Holst (1939) and by the founders of ethology, Konrad Lorenz and Niko Tinbergen. Modern neurobiology has provided extensive experimental evidence for the existence of endogenously generated activity.

The evidence of endogenously generated motility
As early as 1913, Graham-Brown, who worked in Sherrington's laboratory, found that locomotor movements in kittens are not based on reflex activity but on intraspinal generation (Graham-Brown 1913). Erich van Holst spent his experimental life's work on what he called 'Zentrale Automatie' (central automatism) and what is now called the central pattern generator (CPG; see review by Grillner 1999). Well-known examples of CPGs are the central mechanisms for breathing, sucking and chewing, and for locomotion such as swimming, crawling and walking. It is only during the last decade that we have reached a better understanding of the cellular and molecular mechanism responsible for endogenously generated motor activity.

Lower vertebrates especially, such as fish and amphibians, but also mammalian foetuses, have provided good experimental possibilities for exploration of rhythmical patterns. These rhythmical patterns can be generated continuously (e.g. breathing) or episodically (e.g. locomotion), when short or long bouts of rhythmic activity are interspersed with periods of quiescence. The latter arises from active, maintained inhibition of an otherwise rhythmical active network (Staras et al 2003). In addition, there are many non-rhythmical movement patterns, particularly in the human foetus and young infant, which have all the characteristics of being endogenously generated, i.e. without any recognisable external stimulus. Prechtl (1997a) suggested that in these cases the generating neural mechanisms should also be called CPGs, because the relevant motor patterns (e.g. general movements, startles, stretches, yawns) are also clearly constant in form and, therefore, easily recognisable every time they occur (see also review by Forssberg 1999). Their periodical or episodical rate of occurrence, as documented in many actograms of foetal motility (de Vries JIP et al 1985, 1988), pleads for central generation. Even if the theoretical possibility might exist that influences outside the foetus could play a role in generating foetal movements, the striking similarity of actograms of unstimulated low-risk preterm infants at the same postmenstrual age practically excludes such an explanation (Prechtl 1997a).

5

Direct experimental evidence for the central origin of complex and co-ordinated movement patterns comes, of course, only from experiments with developing animals, in which isolated brainstem and spinal cord preparations are studied *in vitro*. Not only do they allow direct extra- or intracellular recordings from various neurons of the CPG network but they also permit the study of transmitters and the use of receptor blockers. In combination with morphological studies, such an approach led to detailed knowledge of the neural mechanism of CPGs and provided an explanation of spontaneous activity. Most CPGs consist, in part, of bistable neurons which generate self-sustaining oscillations of membrane potentials and act as pacemaker-like structures. Isolated CPGs generate fictive locomotor rhythms (recorded in the absence of movements), indicating that the fundamental pattern of motor output depends on the intrinsic connectivity and electrical properties of these central circuits. Sensory inputs are required to modify the pattern of motor activity in response to the actual circumstances of real movement (Suster and Bate 2002).

In the lamprey, the contralaterally alternating ventral root activity is driven by ipsilateral glutamatergic excitation (Buchanan and Grillner 1987) coupled with crossed glycinergic inhibition (Buchanan 1982, Alford and Williams 1989). Glutamatergic excitatory synapses activate AMPA and NMDA receptors known to be necessary for the maintenance of the locomotor rhythm (Takahashi and Alford 2002). Intracellular $Ca2+$, acetylcholine, serotonin, the monoamine precursor L-DOPA, NMDA and AMPA receptors, as well as metabotropic glutamate receptors play an important role (Roberts and Perrins 1995, Spitzer 1995, Antri et al 2002, Cheng et al 2002, Fok and Stein 2002, Navarrete et al 2002, Sadreyev and Panchin 2002, Takahashi and Alford 2002). Presynaptic inhibition and antidromic discharge may have an important role in the control of spontaneous locomotion (Cote and Gossard 2003). In rat foetuses, spontaneously generated activity recorded from ventral roots of lumbar segments is generated by glycine and GABA, which only later act as inhibitory transmitters (Nishimaru et al 1996). In the neonatal rat, the generating network for hindlimb locomotion is located in the first and second lumbar segments, which drives the motoneurons of the lower lumbar segments (Cazalets et al 1995). This highly patterned locomotion even continues if the inhibitory transmitters are pharmacologically blocked (Bracci et al 1996). A differential distribution of phase-specific interneurons is in agreement with observations that revealed distinct but overlapping flexor and extensor centres for walking in the mudpuppy (Cheng et al 2002).

Along the same lines are the extensive studies on the isolated brainstem-spinal cord preparations of the neonatal rat for recording respiratory-like rhythm generation (Suzue 1984, Onimaru 1995). Single unit recordings and pharmacological manipulations clarified the complex nature of the respiratory CPG in the medulla. The extent to which genetic mechanisms are responsible for the production of the respiratory CPG was surveyed by Champagnat and Fortin (1997).

The rich movement repertoire: the continuity from prenatal to postnatal life
Early studies on human foetal movements were carried out on exteriorised foetuses. The survival was limited to a few minutes during which the foetus was stimulated with tactile stimuli (Minkowski 1928, Hooker 1952). These studies remained strictly in the tradition of

reflexology and behaviorism and it is not surprising that the endogenously generated and thus spontaneous activity was totally overlooked or wrongly interpreted. To be fair it should be mentioned that it would hardly have been possible to see spontaneous movements during the short survival time. Today, we know from non-invasive ultrasound observations that these earlier studies described rather abnormal movement patterns of dying foetuses. Moreover, the foetus responded to artificial tactile stimuli, never present in the natural situation (Prechtl 1989b, 2001b).

In the 1980s the breakthrough in foetal movement studies came from the introduction of advanced ultrasound equipment. Prolonged and repeated direct observations became possible. Prechtl and co-workers followed 12 foetuses of carefully selected low-risk pregnancies in weekly intervals from 7 to 8 weeks onwards until 20 weeks and than until term in three- to four-week intervals (de Vries JIP et al 1982, 1984, 1985, 1987, 1988, Prechtl 1989b, 1997b, 1999, 2001b). Another nine foetuses were followed from 28 weeks until term in four-week intervals (Roodenburg et al 1991). Continuous one-hour recordings were made and stored on videotape for off-line analysis.

The first movement to occur is sideward bending of the head. It is first seen at 7½ to 8 weeks postmenstrual age (counted from the first day of the last menstruation before the amenorrhoea). These first movements can clearly be seen by transvaginal transducers (Fig. 2.1) but are poorly detected by transabdominal ultrasound. Time and movement pattern are actually the same as in Hooker's (1952) observation after perioral stimulation with a Frey's hair. Hooker's trigeminal stimulation elicited lateral bending of the head as the first foetal movement due to the newly formed connection of the cervical motor neurons with neck muscles.

At 9 to 10 weeks postmenstrual age, complex and generalised movements occur (de Vries JIP et al 1982, Prechtl 1989b). These are the so-called general movements (Prechtl et al 1979) and the startles. Both include the whole body, but the general movements are slower and have a complex sequence of involved body parts (Fig. 2.2), while the startle is a quick, phasic movement of all limbs, trunk and neck.

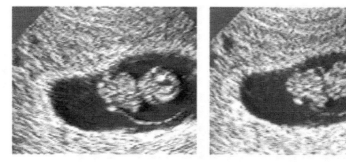

Fig. 2.1 Video prints of first foetal movements observed by transvaginal transducer: sideward bending of the head at 7½ weeks postmenstrual age.

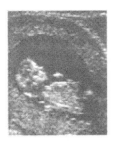

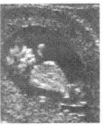

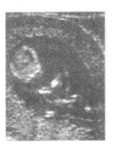

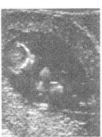

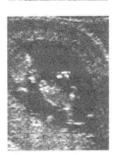

Local and isolated movements of one arm or leg emerge only one week later (at 10 to 11 weeks) than the generalised movements. It may be surmised that isolated movements are more difficult to produce by the very young nervous system than global motor activity. There was another unexpected finding. Traditionally, it is accepted that the early ontogenetic process goes from cranial to caudal. Although this was primarily based on the sensory system (Hooker 1952), the motor system does not follow this rule. Isolated arm and isolated leg movements emerge at the same time, at 10 weeks. However, it is true that isolated arm movements occur more frequently than isolated leg movements, and this might previously have been overlooked in short-lasting recordings (de Vries JIP et al 1982, Prechtl 1989b, 2001b).

Prechtl's observations led to changes of paradigms. In the traditional literature it was assumed that in ontogeny jerky movements precede slow and tonic movements. This is not the case. Tonic and phasic movements emerge at the same age, namely at 9 to 10 weeks postmenstrual age. It may have been that the traditionally short recordings overestimated the more frequent jerky movements and thus led to the wrong conclusion. Along the same lines, it is not true that early movements are random and amorphic followed only later by specific and distinct movements. In fact, all early and later foetal movement patterns are differentiated, right from their very first appearance onwards (Prechtl 1989b, 2001b).

Table 2.1 illustrates the foetal repertoire from 10 weeks postmenstrual age onwards. A striking phenomenon in foetal motor development is the early emergence of stretches and yawns. Both are complex movements and the most interesting aspect is their maintenance throughout the whole life without changing their form and pattern (Prechtl 1989b).

A very important aspect of foetal movements is the change of foetal position *in utero*. Positional changes are frequent and may run up to 25 changes per hour at the end of pregnancy (de Vries JIP et al 1985). Trunk rotations, general movements and alternating leg movements, leading to a somersault if proper contact of the feet can be made with the uterine wall, all produce changes in the intra-uterine position. These motor patterns are obviously an ontogenetic adaptation and have an effective function during prenatal life. The alternating leg movements outlive the duration of pregnancy and are known after birth as the newborn stepping (Prechtl 2001b).

Fig. 2.2 Video print of a foetus (14 weeks postmenstrual age) during general movements.

TABLE 2.1
Foetal motor repertoire (Birnholz 1981, Bots et al 1981, de Vries
JIP et al 1982, Prechtl 1989b). Age is given in postmenstrual weeks

10 weeks	12 weeks	14 weeks	20 weeks
Startle	Startle	Startle	Startle
GMs	GMs	GMs	GMs
Isolated arm ms	Isolated arm ms	Isolated arm ms	Isolated arm ms
Isolated leg ms	Isolated leg ms	Isolated leg ms	Isolated leg ms
Hiccup	Hiccup	Hiccup	Hiccup
	Breathing ms	Breathing ms	Breathing ms
	Hand–face contact	Hand–face contact	Hand–face contact
	Head retroflexion	Head retroflexion	Head retroflexion
	Head anteflexion	Head anteflexion	Head anteflexion
	Head rotation	Head rotation	Head rotation
	Stretch	Stretch	Stretch
	Yawn	Yawn	Yawn
		Sucking and swallowing	Sucking and swallowing
			Eye ms

ms = movements

Breathing movements and eye movements, as well as the sucking and swallowing movements, are anticipating later functions, only becoming effective during postnatal life, and are evidence for the primacy of the motor system. The latter already have a significant intra-uterine function of regulating the amount of amniotic fluid (Prechtl 1989b, 2001b).

There are hardly any changes in the form and pattern of the movements in the first weeks after birth, despite the profound changes in the environmental conditions. Postnatally, some of the endogenously generated motor patterns gradually come under sensory control. Rooting is an outstanding example. In the foetus it is a rhythmical side-to-side head movement and later it becomes directed towards the stimulated peri-oral area (Prechtl 1958). While the foetus drinks amniotic fluid whenever sucking movements occur, after birth sucking behaviour needs to be triggered in the actual feeding situation. Hence, it is a matter of vital biological adaptation that rooting and sucking are elicited in the proper nursing situation initiated by the caregiver. Other examples are postnatal breathing movements and smiling movements (Prechtl 2001b).

New in the motor repertoire after birth are functions depending on the newly installed lung ventilation. Reflexes for protection of the airway such as sneezing and coughing, as well as the communication signal of crying, are only seen after birth (Prechtl 2001b). Prenatally it was not possible to elicit any vestibular responses in the foetus, when the mother had been adequately moved by the experimenter and the foetus simultaneously observed by ultrasound (Prechtl 1997b). However, after birth, vestibular responses such as vestibular-ocular response (von Bernuth and Prechtl 1969, Cioni et al 1984) and the Moro response are clearly present.

By and large, there is an amazing continuation of the prenatal repertoire during the first two months postterm age (Prechtl 1984b, Cioni et al 1989, Hadders-Algra and Prechtl 1992). Needless to say, in the healthy preterm infant this continuation lasts until the same postmenstrual age as in the infant born at term, i.e. the corrected age for preterm birth (Cioni and Prechtl 1990). At around the third month of life a major transformation of many motor and sensory patterns occurs (Prechtl 1984a). This makes the infant more fit to meet the requirements of the extra-uterine environment.

What are general movements?

From the rich repertoire of distinct spontaneous movement patterns the so-called general movements (GMs) are the most frequently occurring and most complex pattern. They are probably what Irwin (1932) called 'mass movements' but he failed to describe these movements more precisely. The term 'general movements' for this specific pattern was coined by Prechtl et al (1979) in an observational study on spontaneous motility in carefully selected low-risk preterm infants. The subsequent foetal studies on the emergence of the different prenatal movement patterns revealed an onset of GMs at 9 weeks postmenstrual age (de Vries JIP et al 1982). They continue to be present during the whole prenatal period (de Vries JIP et al 1985, Prechtl 1989b, Roodenburg et al 1991) until about 5 to 6 months postterm age (Hopkins and Prechtl 1984).

GMs involve the whole body in a variable sequence of arm, leg, neck and trunk movements. They wax and wane in intensity, force and speed, and they have a gradual beginning and end. Rotations along the axis of the limbs and slight changes in the direction of movements make them fluent and elegant and create the impression of complexity and variability (Prechtl 1990).

While before term we call them foetal or preterm GMs, at term age and until about 6 to 9 weeks postterm age, they are called writhing movements (Hopkins and Prechtl 1984). Even if age-related minor differences exist, GMs have by and large a similar appearance from early foetal life until the end of the second month postterm (Fig. 2.3). At 6 to 9 weeks

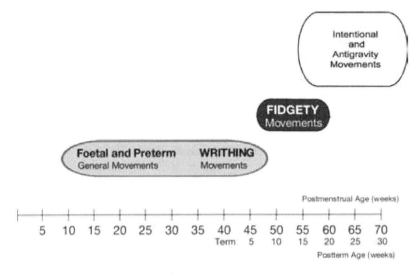

Fig. 2.3 Developmental course of general movements.

10

postterm age, GMs with a writhing character gradually disappear while fidgety GMs gradually emerge (Hopkins and Prechtl 1984, Prechtl et al 1997a). Fidgety movements are present up to the end of the first half-year of life when intentional and antigravity movements occur and start to dominate (Fig. 2.3).

PRETERM GMs
No difference can be observed between foetal and preterm GMs, indicating that neither the increase of the force of gravity after birth nor maturation has an influence on the appearance of GMs. The GMs of a preterm infant may occasionally have large amplitudes and are often of fast speed (Cioni and Prechtl 1990; see Fig. 2.4 and Cases A and B on the DVD).

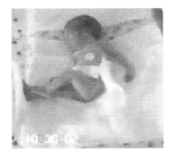

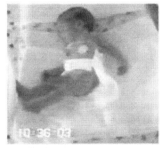

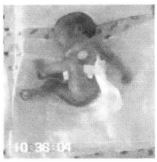

WRITHING MOVEMENTS
At term age and during the first two months postterm, GMs are commonly referred to as writhing movements (Hopkins and Prechtl 1984, Prechtl and Hopkins 1986, Cioni et al 1989, Cioni and Prechtl 1990, Prechtl et al 1997a). They are characterised by small to moderate amplitude and by slow to moderate speed. Typically, they are ellipsoid in form, which creates the impression of a writhing quality (see Fig. 2.5 and Case C on the DVD).

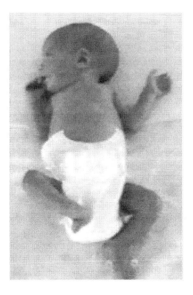

Fig. 2.4 Three-second sequence (36:02 to 36:04) of GMs with large amplitude in a preterm infant, aged 34 weeks (Case B on the DVD).

Fig. 2.5 Fullterm neonate with writhing movements (Case C on the DVD).

EMG recordings revealed that the burst duration was significantly longer during preterm GMs than during writhing movements. However, burst amplitude values and tonic background data do not change from preterm GMs to GMs of writhing quality (Hadders-Algra and Prechtl 1993).

At 6 to 9 weeks postterm age, writhing movements gradually disappear while fidgety GMs gradually emerge (Hopkins and Prechtl 1984, Cioni and Prechtl 1990, Hadders-Algra and Prechtl 1992, Prechtl et al 1997a).

FIDGETY MOVEMENTS

At the time of the major neural transformation (see Chapter 1) the fidgety type of GM appears (Hopkins and Prechtl 1984). Fidgety movements are small movements of moderate speed and variable acceleration, of neck, trunk and limbs, in all directions, continual in the awake infant, except during fussing and crying (see Fig. 2.6 and Cases D to F on the DVD; Prechtl et al 1997a, 1997b). They may be seen as early as 6 weeks but usually occur around 9 weeks and are present until 20 weeks (Prechtl et al 1997b) or even a few weeks longer, at which time intentional and antigravity movements occur and start to dominate. An early onset of fidgety movements (around 6 weeks) can mainly be observed in infants born preterm (Cioni and Prechtl 1990).

EMG characteristics change with age (Fig. 2.7). Phasic burst duration shortens progressively with increasing age. The amplitude of the phasic bursts and the tonic background activity decrease during the transformation from writhing to fidgety movements. What both GM characters have in common is the variation in onset of muscle activity and the large amount of co-activation (up to 80 per cent) in antagonistic muscle groups (Hadders-Algra et al 1992, Hadders-Algra 1993, Hadders-Algra et al 1997).

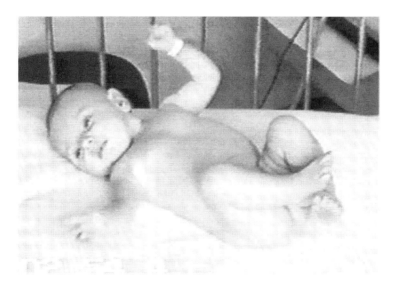

Fig. 2.6 Three-month-old infant with fidgety movements (Case D on the DVD).

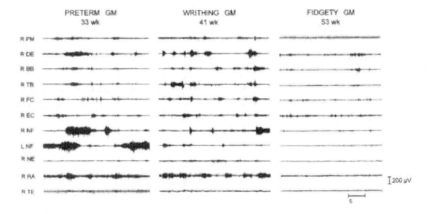

Fig. 2.7 EMG pattern of normal GMs in a 33-week-old preterm infant (left); writhing GMs at 1 week postterm age (middle); and fidgety movements at 13 weeks postterm age (right) (reproduced with permission from Hadders-Algra et al 1997).

L = left, R = right, PM = pectoralis major, DE = deltoid muscle, BB = biceps brachii, TB = triceps brachii, FC = flexor carpi, EC = extensor carpi, NF = neck flexor, RA = rectus abdominis, TE = thoracic extensor

The main kinematic aspects of the transformation from writhing to fidgety movements can also be seen by means of 3-D-motion analysis. Coluccini et al (2002) have studied the distribution of movement velocity and amplitude of GMs in a group of healthy fullterm infants recorded from 7 to 12 weeks of age. A clear decrease of movement velocity and amplitude was observed (Fig. 2.8).

The temporal organisation of fidgety movements varies with age. Initially, they occur as isolated events (score: + or +/–, Fig. 2.8, middle graph); they gradually increase in frequency (score: ++, Fig. 2.8 bottom graph) and then decrease once again (score: + or +/–) (Prechtl et al 1997a, 1997b). This temporal organisation can be defined as follows (Dibiasi and Einspieler 2002).

Continual fidgety movements (score: ++)
Fidgety movements occur frequently but are interspersed with short pauses. As fidgety movements are by definition GMs, the movements involve the whole body, particularly the neck, trunk, shoulders, wrists, hips and ankles. Depending on the actual body posture, in particular the position of the head, fidgety movements may be expressed differently in the different body parts.

Intermittent fidgety movements (score: +)
Although fidgety movements occur regularly in all body parts, the temporal organisation differs from fidgety movements ++. In fact, the pauses between fidgety movements are prolonged, giving the impression that fidgety movements are present for only half of the observation time.

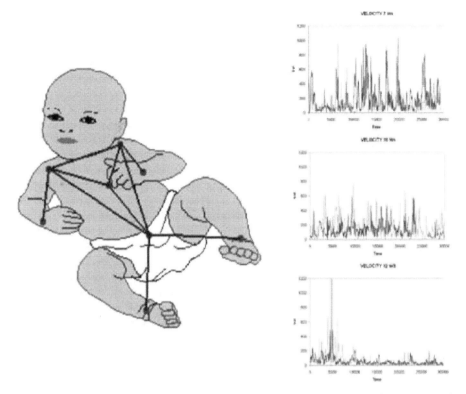

Fig. 2.8 3-D motion analysis of GMs in a normal infant recorded at 7, 10 and 12 weeks postterm age by means of an opto-electronic system (ELITE 2002, BTS Milan, Italy). Reflective markers were applied at the level of dorsal surface of each hand and foot, at the shoulders, sternum and pubis. Kinematic data have been synchronised with simultaneous digital video recording of the movements. The graphs reporting the velocity traces (mm/sec in the y-axis) of the markers placed in the right ■ and left ▨ hand during a 30-second period of time indicate a clear increase of slower distal movements, from writhing GMs at 7 weeks (top graph), to intermittent fidgety movements (score +) at 10 weeks (middle graph) and continual fidgety movements (score ++) at 12 weeks (bottom graph). At 12 weeks occasional high velocity movements are superimposed.

Sporadic fidgety movements (score: +/-)
Sporadic fidgety movements are like fidgety movements + but interspersed with even longer pauses.

Fidgety movements are usually equally present in the distal (D) and proximal (P) body parts (score: D = P). However, there are some infants with more fidgety activity in the wrists and ankles than in the trunk and proximal joints. These fidgety movements are scored D > P. If fidgety movements are more prominent in the neck, trunk, shoulders and hips, we score this P > D. This differentiation seems relevant for the prediction of a less optimal neurological outcome (see Chapter 5).

In 3- to 6-month-old infants various other movements may occur together with fidgety

14

movements, such as wiggling-oscillating and saccadic arm movements, swipes, mutual manipulation of fingers, manipulation (fiddling) of clothing, reaching and touching, legs lift with or without hand–knee contact, trunk rotation, and axial rolling (Fig. 2.9 and Table 2.2). Fidgety movements are superimposed on other movements, or other movements may occur during the pauses between fidgety movements, or both.

General movements are most probably generated supraspinally

To our knowledge, no studies exist, not even in animal experiments, which address the generation of startles or GMs. As both movement types include activity of all segments from cervical to lumbar spinal cord, it is likely that the generating neuronal structure is

TABLE 2.2
Movement patterns, which may occur together with fidgety movements (Hopkins and Prechtl 1984, Cioni and Prechtl 1990, Hadders-Algra and Prechtl 1992, Einspieler 1994, Prechtl 2001b)

Movement pattern	Definition	Period of occurrence
Wiggling-oscillating arm movements	Irregular, oscillatory, waving-like movements; most noticeable in partially or fully extended arms, where they have a frequency of 2 to 3 Hz; small amplitude and moderate speed; should be clearly distinguished from tremulous movements, which are less smooth in appearance and have a more regular rhythm	6 to 14 weeks postterm age
Saccadic arm movements	Jerky, zigzag movements, which continually vary in direction; most noticeable in partially or fully extended arms; moderate to large amplitude and moderate speed	6 to 15 weeks postterm age
Swiping movements	Movements with a sudden but fluid onset and smooth offset with a ballistic-like appearance; can go in downward or upward direction; most noticeable in extended arms, but also in partially or fully extended legs; large amplitude and high speed	6 to 20 weeks postterm age
Mutual manipulation of fingers	Both hands are brought together in the midline and the fingers of both hands repetitively touch, stroke or grasp each other	From 12 weeks postterm age onwards
Manipulation (fiddling) of clothing	The fingers of one or both hands repetitively touch, stroke or grasp some object or the clothing	From 12 weeks postterm age onwards
Reaching and touching	One or both arms extend to some object in the immediate environment. The fingers contact the surface of the object	From 12 weeks postterm age onwards
Legs lift	Both legs lift vertically upward; partial or full extension at the knees; hips are slightly tilted upward; one or both hands touching or grasping the knees; sometimes with anteflexion of the head	From 15 weeks postterm age onwards
Trunk rotation	As a result of the soles of the feet pushing down on the lying surface, one side of the hips is lifted and rotated	From 12 weeks postterm age onwards
Axial rolling	The whole body is turned from supine to prone lying in a movement started by the head. Sometimes the infant returns to prone lying	From 18 weeks postterm age onwards

15

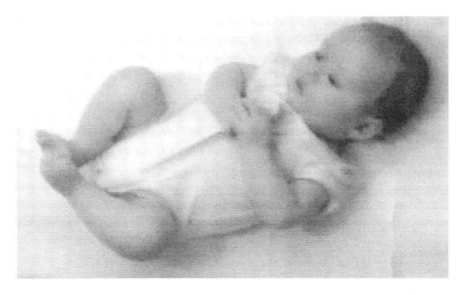

Fig. 2.9 Fourteen-week-old infant with fidgety movements, mutual hand contact with fiddling, and mutual feet contact.

located supraspinally (Prechtl 1997a). Both movements emerge in the human foetus at 9 to 10 weeks postmenstrual age, which makes it unlikely that higher structures than the brainstem are involved. It can also be assumed that GMs of writhing quality and those of fidgety quality are generated by different CPGs. Their temporal overlap at the transformation from the one type into the other makes this most plausible (Prechtl 1997a). That writhing movements do not disappear during sleep even at 6 months is indicative of the prolonged preservation of their CPG during the fidgety movement period and thereafter (Einspieler et al 1994).

Alternating leg movements in foetuses, which are involved in the frequent changes of the intra-uterine position, have a CPG with low spinal localisation. The research on anencephalic foetuses included one case in which only the low thoracic and lumbar spinal cord was normally organised (Visser et al 1985). The more cranial structures were lacking or severely abnormal. This foetus generated excessive alternating leg movements, never seen in an intact foetus. The CPG of this rhythmical activity must, therefore, have existed in this limited spinal structure (Prechtl 1997a).

General movements change their quality if the nervous system is impaired
The quality of GMs is probably modulated by more cranial structures (e.g. cortico-spinal, reticulo-spinal) and hence can be affected by impairments of these structures. A disruption of the cortico-spinal projections by periventricular lesions of the corona radiata or internal capsule due to haemorrhages or hypoxic-ischaemic lesions (leukomalacia) leads to abnormal GMs. According to PET (positron emission tomography) scan data the sensori-motor cortex is already active in the neonate (Chugani and Phelps 1986, Chugani et al 1987). On the

16

other hand, behavioural evidence for functional activity of these cortical areas in the form of voluntary movements and differentiated isolated finger movements is lacking at this age. This is even more evident at preterm age. Despite these facts we must consider a modulating influence of these cortico-spinal connections on the GM-CPGs (Prechtl 1997a). Cortico-spinal fibres were found in the human foetus at the cervical segments as early as 16 weeks postmenstrual age (Okado and Kojima 1984). Their synaptic input on lower segments can be expected at preterm and term age.

If the nervous system is impaired, GMs lose their complex and variable character and have a poor repertoire, or are cramped-synchronised or chaotic. This holds true for the preterm, term and early postterm age (first two months). Fidgety movements can be either abnormal or absent.

POOR REPERTOIRE GMs
This abnormal GM pattern occurs during preterm, term and early postterm age. The sequence of the successive movement components is monotonous and movements of the different body parts do not occur in the complex way seen in normal GMs (Ferrari et al 1990, Einspieler et al 1997; Cases G and H on the DVD). Poor repertoire GMs are frequent in infants with brain ultrasound abnormalities and can be followed by normal, abnormal or absent fidgety movement. Hence, the predictive value is rather low (Prechtl et al 1997b).

CRAMPED-SYNCHRONISED GMs
This is an abnormal pattern from preterm age onwards. Movements appear rigid and lack the normal smooth and fluent character; all limb and trunk muscles contract and relax almost simultaneously (Ferrari et al 1990, Einspieler et al 1997; Cases J and K on the DVD). If this abnormal pattern is observed consistently over a number of weeks it is of high predictive value for the development of spastic cerebral palsy (Ferrari et al 1990, Prechtl et al 1997b, Ferrari et al 2002; see also Chapter 5).

CHAOTIC GMs
Movements of all limbs are of large amplitude and occur in a chaotic order without any fluency or smoothness. They consistently appear to be abrupt (Bos et al 1997b, Einspieler et al 1997, Ferrari et al 1997; Case L on the DVD). Chaotic GMs can be observed during preterm, term and early postterm age but are rather rare. Infants with chaotic GMs often develop cramped-synchronised GMs a few weeks later.

ABNORMAL FIDGETY MOVEMENTS
These look like normal fidgety movements but their amplitude, speed and jerkiness are moderately or greatly exaggerated (Prechtl et al 1997b; Case M on the DVD). Abnormal fidgety movements are rare. Their predictive value is low (Prechtl et al 1997b; see also Chapter 5).

ABSENCE OF FIDGETY MOVEMENTS

If fidgety movements are never observed from 9 to 20 weeks postterm we call this abnormality 'absence of fidgety movements' (Cases N and O on the DVD). Other movements can, however, be commonly observed (Prechtl et al 1997b). The absence of fidgety movements is highly predictive for later neurological impairments, particularly for cerebral palsy, both the spastic (Prechtl et al 1997b) and dyskinetic forms (Einspieler et al 2002; see also Chapter 5). If the cramped-synchronised character is still present at 3 to 4 months (or even longer), fidgety movements are absent (Case O on the DVD).

3
HOW TO RECORD AND ASSESS GENERAL MOVEMENTS

The simplest way of assessing motor activity is by directly observing the movements with the unaided eye. However, considerable improvement in the reliability of the assessment is achieved if the infant's GMs are observed by replaying a video recording. There is the advantage of repeated playback, including at different speeds, and of storing the recordings for documentation and future reference.

Recording technique

In order to provide a reliable assessment of GMs the recording procedure has to be standardised and certain behavioural states, such as crying, are not suitable for an assessment.

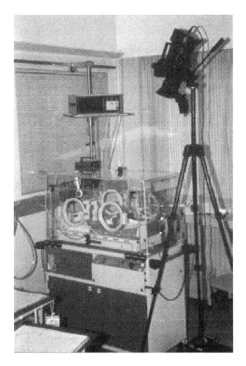

Fig. 3.1 Video recording of a preterm infant in the incubator; the camera is placed high above the infant on a tripod.

EQUIPMENT

The video camera should be placed high above the infant (Fig. 3.1). In order to keep the older infant's attention to the camera to a minimum a small camera is preferable. A single-chip camera does not even have a blinking light during recording. In our experience, it is not necessary to use a camera hidden above a purpose-built bed surrounded by white curtains, as mentioned by Geerdink and Hopkins (1993a), as the infant quickly habituates to the camera. Very attractive objects may interfere with the temporal organisation of fidgety movements, but this will not last more than 20 to 30 seconds (Dibiasi and Einspieler 2002, see Chapter 4). Digital cameras are preferable. For the selection of GMs from the recording and the subsequent analysis, a time code signal superimposed on the tape is helpful.

Watching a monitor outside the observation room is a useful way of observing the infant without causing interference. In

19

this way, parents can be asked to soothe their baby if it starts crying because then the recording must be interrupted anyway.

PROCEDURE

Depending on its age the infant should lie in a supine position in the incubator, bed or on a mattress on the floor. Recording infants lying on a table or baby-dressing table should be avoided for the infant's safety. The caregiver's presence will not only attract the infant's attention but also interfere with the observer's Gestalt perception. The observer must be able to see the infant's face to make sure that rigid movements are not due to crying. This is especially important as the later assessment is done without acoustic signals.

A small and non-restrictive nappy is advisable. In very young preterm infants we usually open the nappy in order to avoid restriction of leg movements (Fig. 3.2). During the postterm period infants should be dressed lightly and comfortably, leaving arms and legs bare (Fig. 3.3). The room temperature should be comfortable, fitting the infant's age and clothing. If the ambient temperature is either too low or too high it will affect the infant's behavioural state and the movement quality.

Most important for the assessment of GM quality is the correct behavioural state (Einspieler et al 1997). However, behavioural states are not established before about 36 weeks postmenstrual age (Nijhuis et al 1982). In infants older than 36 weeks recordings should preferably be performed during state 4 (Einspieler et al 1997), which is characterised by open eyes, irregular respiration, present movements, and absent crying (active wakefulness; Prechtl 1974). Younger preterm infants should be recorded when bouts of activity

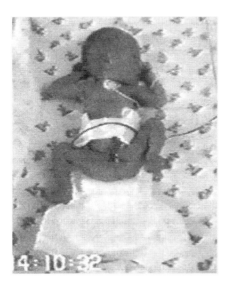

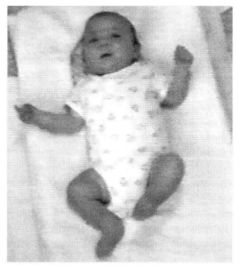

Fig. 3.2 For the GM assessment the preterm infant's nappy is partly opened and only closed above the belly.

Fig. 3.3 During the postterm period the infant should be dressed lightly and comfortably, leaving arms and legs bare.

occur, irrespective of whether the infant is awake or sleeping (Einspieler et al 1997). The same holds true for infants older than 36 weeks with severe brain lesion as their behavioural states may be profoundly disorganised (Prechtl 1974).

The duration of the recording depends on the age of the infant. In order to collect about three GMs for a reliable assessment we usually record preterm infants for 30 to 60 minutes. This does not require the observer's presence during the recording nor the later assessment of the whole recording. Preferably, the recording should be started by the staff of the neonatal unit, provided it does not interfere with nursing. Such a long recording ensures sufficient activity bouts on tape. Later, this recording is viewed at fast speed and about three GM sequences are copied onto the assessment tape.

From the writhing movement period onwards, five to ten minutes of optimal recording is usually sufficient. It is helpful if the sequential recordings of the infant, taken at different ages, are stored on a separate assessment tape for the documentation of the individual developmental course.

WHAT SHOULD BE AVOIDED?
As GMs are dependent on the behavioural state (Prechtl 1990, Hadders-Algra et al 1993, Einspieler et al 1994, 1997), the movements change during fussing, crying and drowsiness. Therefore, the recording should not be continued during prolonged episodes of fussing and crying or during drowsiness. Nor is it possible to judge the quality of GMs properly if the infant is sucking on a dummy. Soothing the infant with a dummy results in the sucking posture (Prechtl and Lenard 1968) with flexed arms, fisting, and extended legs (Fig. 3.4).

In cases of prolonged fussing and crying the recording must be stopped. Only restart the recording after the infant has been soothed. This may take some time. It may even be necessary to repeat the recording session on another day. However, it should be mentioned

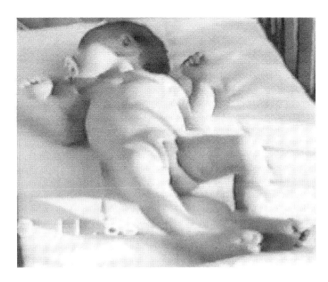

Fig. 3.4 Sucking on a dummy results in the sucking posture. GM assessment is no longer possible.

that infants with severe brain dysfunction may frequently cry after they start moving, e.g. infants with cramped-synchronised GMs.

Prolonged episodes of hiccuping should not be assessed. They interfere with the GMs as well as with the observer's Gestalt perception.

Interference by an observer (parent, examiner) and the presence of toys in the immediate vicinity should be avoided. Although we know that spontaneous movements are quite stable and robust and hardly interfered with by stimulation (Dibiasi and Einspieler 2002; see also Chapter 4), the observer's Gestalt perception might be destroyed by too many distracting objects or persons (Fig. 3.5). The same applies for a mattress covered by a colourful patterned blanket (Fig. 3.6).

We certainly advise against putting the infant in front of a mirror, which is sometimes used in recording or treatment rooms. The mirror image, acting as a 'twin', destroys the observer's Gestalt perception. In addition, older infants are attracted by their 'twin', touching the mirror and smiling towards it.

Finally, we advise against recording GMs during the first three days after birth. During these early days, many physiological variables tend to fluctuate more than they do later. There is also an initial instability of behavioural states, changing rapidly from quiet sleep to crying, which can interfere with a proper observation of GMs. It is therefore advisable to avoid this period of instability if not otherwise indicated.

Visual Gestalt perception as a scientific tool for general movement analysis

Gestalt perception is a powerful instrument in the analysis of complex phenomena. In his paper 'Gestalt perception as a source of scientific knowledge' the Nobel prize laureate Konrad Lorenz pointed out that 'Gestalt perception is able to take into account a greater number of individual details and more relationships between these than in any rational calculation' (Lorenz 1971). Visual Gestalt perception is used whenever dynamic or static images are globally assessed. Pattern recognition is employed in this procedure.

In a time of ever more technical diagnostic procedures, old-fashioned direct observation is lost or is, at least, treated with disrespect as a subjective method. As soon as a machine is between the patient and the examiner, the method is considered as 'objective'. It tends to be forgotten that visual analysis of an X-ray picture, an EEG recording, MRI pictures, etc., is also based on visual Gestalt perception and is no more objective than straightforward observation with the unaided eye, analysing video recordings of movement patterns (Accardo 1997, Prechtl 2001a).

The average interscorer agreement of the qualitative assessment of GMs in a number of studies on several hundred infants was more than 90 per cent (Einspieler et al 1997, Valentin, personal communication). Details on interscorer agreement are provided in Chapter 5.

In applying the visual Gestalt perception to the assessment of GMs, the first step is to differentiate between normal GMs and abnormal GMs. If GMs are considered to be abnormal the different age-specific sub-categories are classified as: poor repertoire GMs, chaotic GMs, cramped-synchronised GMs, abnormal fidgety movements, absence of fidgety movements (for definitions, see Chapter 2).

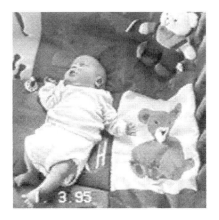

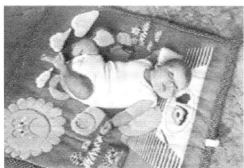

Fig. 3.5 Video print of a 2-week-old infant: too many toys might interfere with the observer's Gestalt perception during GM assessment.

Fig. 3.6 Video print of a 7-week-old infant: a colourful blanket might impair the visual Gestalt perception and makes GM assessment difficult.

During the video analysis of the GM quality, environmental interference must be avoided. This includes doing the assessment without acoustic signals. In addition, other caregivers, siblings or twins, mirror images of the infant, a bed crowded with toys (Fig. 3.5), or an irritating coloured blanket (Fig. 3.6) on the video all impair the observer's Gestalt perception.

As tiredness interferes with the visual Gestalt perception, the observer should never assess for longer periods than about 45 minutes without taking a break.

If many recordings of abnormal GMs are seen in a series it is advisable to watch a criterion standard normal recording from time to time. This is necessary for re-calibrating the Gestalt perception. The examples on the enclosed DVD should be at hand for this purpose.

Individual developmental trajectories based on longitudinal recordings
The results of most follow-up studies provide only a statistical chance that an individual will eventually develop a particular impairment, relative to a low-risk reference group. A somewhat different approach seemed advisable (Prechtl 1990). When the quality of GMs is repeatedly assessed during the preterm, term and postterm period until about 20 weeks, an individual developmental trajectory can be obtained indicating the consistency or inconsistency of normal or abnormal findings (Prechtl 1990). Individuals with similar trajectories can be grouped, which improves the specific prediction of the individual outcome. A snapshot assessment of a single recording must be avoided. An individual developmental trajectory should document the following GM assessments:

- two to three recordings of the preterm period (three GM sequences each)
- one recording at term or early postterm age or both

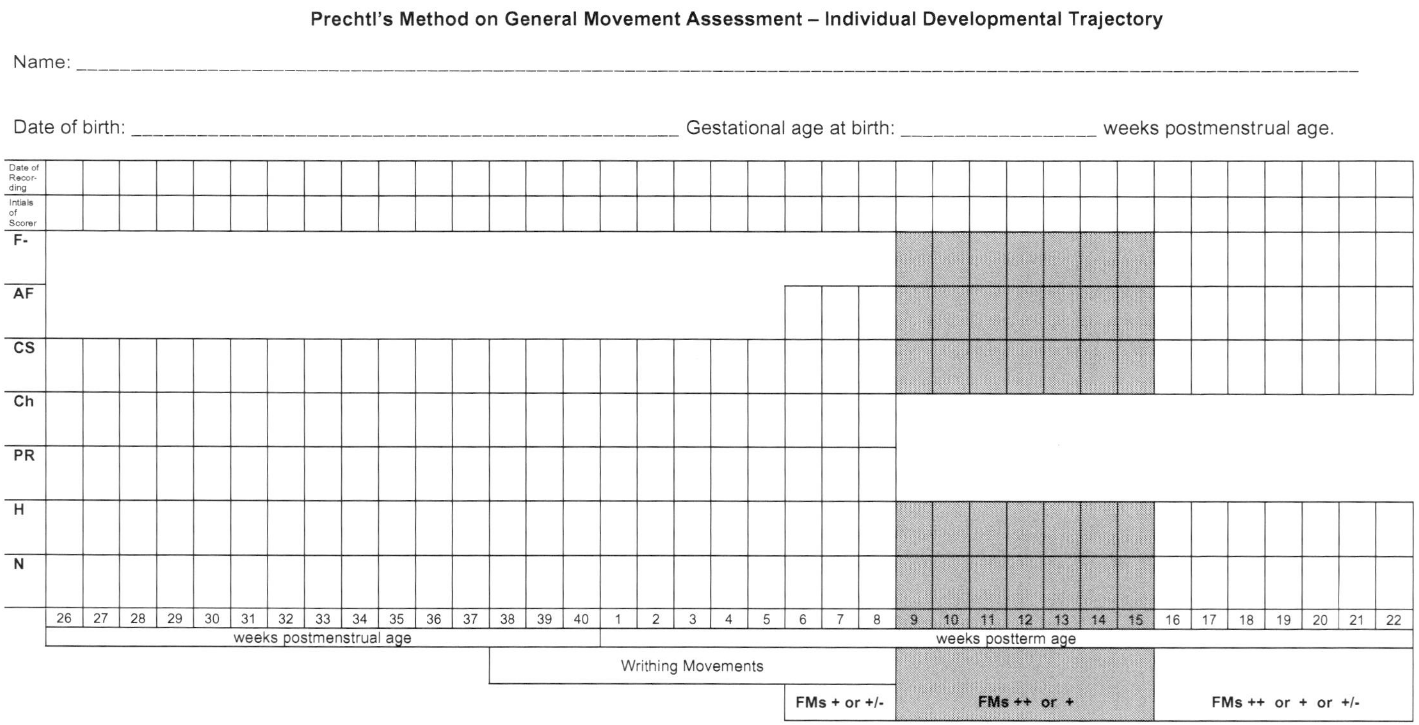

Prechtl's Method on General Movement Assessment – Individual Developmental Trajectory

Name: _____

Date of birth: _____   Gestational age at birth: _____   weeks postmenstrual age.

| Date of Recording | | | | | | | | | | | | | | | | | | | | | | | | | | | | | |
| Initials of Scorer | | | | | | | | | | | | | | | | | | | | | | | | | | | | | |

weeks postmenstrual age: 26 27 28 29 30 31 32 33 34 35 36 37 38 39 40 | 1 2 3 4 5 6 7 8 9 10 11 12 13 14 15 16 17 18 19 20 21 22 weeks postterm age

Rows: F-, AF, CS, Ch, PR, H, N

Writhing Movements | Fidgety Movements

FMs + or +/-

FMs ++ or +

FMs ++ or + or +/-

N, normal age-specific GMs; FMs, fidgety movements; H, hypokinesis (no GMs during the recording); PR, poor repertoire of GMs; Ch, chaotic GMs; CS, cramped-synchronised GMs; AF, abnormal fidgety movements; F-, absence of fidgety movements. The shaded area indicates the age period during which fidgety movements usually occur.

Fig. 3.7 Proforma for the individual developmental trajectory.

24

- at least one recording between 9 and 15 weeks postterm. If an absence of fidgety movements is found the infant should be recorded a second time during the fidgety movement period, e.g. at 12 and 15 weeks postterm age

Fig. 3.7 provides the proforma of the individual developmental trajectory. The design of this proforma is related to the findings on the predictive value of GM assessment (see Chapter 5). The more often and the earlier the individual developmental trajectory deviates from the bottom line the higher is the probability for the development of neurological deficits. In addition, the individual developmental trajectory documents deterioration or improvement of GMs at particular ages.

Two age-specific motor optimality scores for semi-quantitative assessment
After the global judgement, it can be worthwhile to look at different aspects and components of GMs, particularly if they are abnormal. A semi-quantification of the GM quality can be achieved by applying Prechtl's optimality concept (Prechtl 1980). For every movement criterion such as amplitude, speed, movement character, sequence, range in space, onset and offset of GMs, a score for optimal or non-optimal performance is given. Thus, the higher the total optimality score the better is the quality of the GMs.

Because of the age-specific character of GMs (see Chapter 2), two different optimality scoring lists are necessary. The first scoring list (Fig. 3.8) is concerned with preterm and

Prechtl's Method on General Movement Assessment
GM Optimality List for Preterm GMs and Writhing Movements
(Ferrari et al 1990, modified)

Name: _____

Date of birth: _____ Gestational age at birth: _____ weeks
Recording date: _____ Recording age: _____ weeks

1. Quality	normal, variable, complex	.4
	poor repertoire	.2
	chaotic	.1
	cramped-synchronised	.1
2. Sequence	variable	.2
	monotonous within GM	.1
	similar from GM to GM	.1
	disorganised	.1
3. Amplitude	variable, full range	.2
	predominantly small range	.1
	predominantly large range	.1
	mainly one range, not variable	.1
4. Speed	variable	.2
	monotonously slow	.1
	monotonously fast	.1
	mainly one speed, not variable	.1
5. Space	from horizontal to vertical plane	.2
	not the full space used	.1
6. Rotatory components	present, fluent and elegant	.2
	no or just a few rotations	.1
7. Onset and offset	smooth	.2
	minimal fluctuations or abrupt	.1
8. Tremulous movements	absent	.2
	present	.1

GM Optimality Score:_____ Maximum: 16; Minimum: 8.

Fig. 3.8 Proforma for the GM optimality score (preterm and writhing GMs).

25

Assessment of Motor Repertoire - 3 to 5 Months
Christa Einspieler and Arie Bos, the GM Trust 2001

Name: ....

born: .... Postmenstrual Age: .... Birth weight: ....

Recording Date: .... Postterm Age: ....

Number of movement patterns observed: ⊔⊔ normal (N) ⊔⊔ abnormal (A)

N A fidgety movements	N	hand-face contact	N A	legs lift, flexion at knees	
N A swiping movements	N	hand-mouth contact	N A	legs lift extension at knees	
N A wiggling-oscillating movem.	N	hand-hand contact	N	hand-knee contact	
N A saccadic arm movements	N	hand-hand manipulation	N A	arching	
N A kicking	N A	fiddling / clothes, blanket	N A	trunk rotation	
N A excitement bursts	N	reaching	N	axial rolling	
A 'cha-cha-cha movements'	N A	foot-foot contact	N A	visual scanning	
N A smiles	N	foot-foot manipulation	N	hand regard	
N A mouth movements	N A	segmental movements arms	N	head anteflexion	
N A tongue movements	N A	segmental movements legs		A arm movements in circles	
N A head rotation	N A	segm: discrepancy arm-leg		A almost no leg movements	

Number of postural patterns observed: ⊔⊔ normal (N) ⊔⊔ abnormal (A)

N A head in midline (20°)	N	variable finger postures	A	hyperextension of the neck
N A symmetrical	A	predominant fisting	A	hyperextension of trunk
N A spontaneous ATNR absent or could be overcome	A	finger spreading	A	extended arms/ on / above surface are predominant
A body and limbs 'flat' on surface	A	few finger postures	A	extended legs / on / above surface are predominant
	A	synchronised opening and closing of the fingers		

Movement character (global score)

N smooth and fluent	A stiff	A predominantly slow speed	
A jerky	A cramped	A predominantly fast speed	
A monotonous	A synchronous	A predomin. large amplitude	
A tremulous	A cramped-synchronised	A predomin. small amplitude	

Motor Optimality List

1.	Fidgety Movements	normal	❑	12
		abnormal	❑	4
	± + ++ P D	absent	❑	1
2.	Repertoire of co-existent other movements	age-adequate	❑	4
		reduced	❑	2
		absent	❑	1
3.	Quality of other movements	N > A	❑	4
		N = A	❑	2
		N < A	❑	1
4.	Posture	N > A	❑	4
		N = A	❑	2
		N < A	❑	1
5.	Movement character	smooth and fluent	❑	4
		abnormal, not cramped-synchr.	❑	2
		cramped-synchronised	❑	1

Motor Optimality Score:
Maximum: 28; Minimum: 5

Fig. 3.9 Proforma for the assessment of the motor repertoire of 3- to 5-month-old infants.

term age (adapted from Ferrari et al 1990). The movement sequence (item 2) is never optimal in abnormal GMs. However, amplitude (item 3) and speed (item 4) might be less optimal even in GMs judged as normal. The second scoring list (Fig. 3.9) covers the motor behaviour of 3- to 6-month-old infants.

An obvious limitation of such a detailed scoring is that this procedure does not allow a re-synthesis from the description of the details to the total picture. With this semi-quantitative approach (which focuses on details) the power of the global Gestalt perception is lost. However, it is helpful to semi-quantitatively describe any change in the quality of GMs, assessing either improvement or worsening during the developmental course.

For the definitions of the specific movement patterns see Chapter 2 (Table 2.2). Segmental movements and arm movements in circles are described in Chapter 5.

Score the following movement patterns abnormal if:

- fidgety movements are absent or of abnormal quality;
- swipes are predominant;
- wiggling-oscillating movements are predominant;
- saccadic arm movements are predominant;
- kicking is monotonous;
- excitement bursts are monotonous and predominant without pleasure mimic;
- 'cha-cha-cha movements' (the abbreviation is not related to the dance) are abnormal excitement burst-like movements: brisk, not elegant, monotonous, if not stereotyped; limb accelerations in all directions; movements towards the midline are lacking; they are ongoing in the whole body and not related to facial expression of excitement;
- smiles are frozen;
- mouth movements are synchronously opening and closing;
- tongue protrusion is repetitive or long-lasting;
- head rotation is repetitive;
- fiddling is awkward;
- foot–foot contact is without small movements and mainly on tibial side;
- segmental movements are side dominant or only present in either upper or lower extremities;
- legs lift with flexion at knees is without variation;
- legs lift with extension at knees is predominant and of stiff character;
- arching is prolonged;
- trunk rotation is *en bloc*;
- visual scanning consists of rowing eye movements.

Score the following postural patterns abnormal if:

- head is only in lateral position (more than 20° from the midline);
- posture is asymmetrical;
- spontaneous ATNR cannot be overcome by the flexion of the jaw arm.

For the age-adequate repertoire (item 2) see Chapter 2 (Table 2.2).

In addition, a GM optimality score can be used for statistical calculations and comparisons with other measurements, as has been done by Einspieler (1994). She reported a high correlation between the GM optimality score and the p02-values obtained during overnight polygraphies in 3- to 20-week-old infants, indicating that drops in p02 resulted in a less optimal GM performance.

4

WHAT COULD INTERFERE WITH THE QUALITY OF GENERAL MOVEMENTS?

Developmental care for preterm infants

Individualised developmental care in the neonatal intensive care unit (NICU) focuses on postural care (mainly by putting preterm infants into a 'nest') and on minimising distressing factors for the infant. It has positive effects on the stability of some physiological indexes, on the number of days of ventilatory support, the duration of hospitalisation and the rate of weight gain (Stevens et al 1996, Brown and Heermann 1997).

Recently, the GMs of two groups of high-risk preterm infants matched for clinical characteristics were compared (Baldi 2002). One group was submitted to conventional care and the second to an individualised developmental care programme. The frequency of normal, poor repertoire, cramped-synchronised and chaotic GMs was the same in both groups. A slight reduction on some indexes of neonatal distress (such as number of startles during wakefulness, number and duration of crying episodes) was observed in the infants submitted to developmental care. More controlled studies are necessary in this field.

Skin-to-skin holding, also known as kangaroo care, has been shown to be beneficial for the preterm infant. In order to investigate an eventual change of rest–activity cycles the occurrence of GMs as a marker of activity level has been studied (Constantinou et al 1999). However, the percentage of GMs did not differ as a result of skin-to-skin holding.

These studies indicate that GMs, being endogenously generated and a robust output of the young nervous system, are hardly influenced by environmental stimulation. For the recording and GM assessment session, however, it is better to take the infant out of the nest because of possible mechanical restriction.

Is general movement assessment under intensive care conditions possible?

In contrast to a neurological examination, GM assessment can be carried out even under intensive care conditions (Albers and Jorch 1994). It is a great advantage that GM assessment is carried out without any handling of the infant and the infant is not even touched (Prechtl 1990). Artificial ventilation, infusion lines (Fig. 4.1) and electrodes allow GM assessment as long as the infant can and does move.

During these very early days after birth the GM assessment might mainly be used to determine acute neurological dysfunction and eventually to evaluate possible effects of medication and intervention. It is not primarily used to predict later neurological outcome.

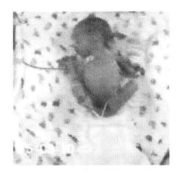

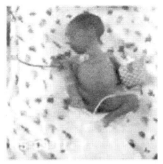

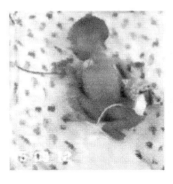

Fig. 4.1 29-week-old preterm infant: despite infusion lines the left arm moves from flexion to extension with a superimposed rotation (from Case A on the DVD).

Effect of drugs on general movement quality

BARBITURATES

No systematic studies on the effect of barbiturates on GMs are available. Ten years ago, Prechtl et al (1993) described how fullterm neonates with hypoxic-ischaemic encephalopathy are hypokinetic during their first days or even a few weeks after birth. All of them were under barbiturate treatment. However, four infants with mild asphyxia had received a comparable dosis of phenobarbitone but were not hypokinetic.

ANTICONVULSANT THERAPY DURING PREGNANCY

Antiepileptic drug therapy (valproic acid, phenobarbital, carbamazepine, lamotrigine, primidone) may have an impact on the course of pregnancy and pregnancy outcome, and may also induce effects on the developing brain that only appear later in life (Scolnik et al 1994, Ornoy and Cohen 1996, Parisi et al 2003). A recent study on eleven cases demonstrated that the optimality scores for GMs (according to the score list: see Fig. 3.8) at 7 days and 4 weeks were markedly reduced. Furthermore, the lower the GM optimality score, the lower the Brunet–Lezine (1967) Developmental Quotient at 30 months (Parisi et al 2003).

INDOMETHACIN

Indomethacin is widely used for non-invasive closure of patent ductus arteriosus in preterm infants (Clyman 1996). In addition, low-dose indomethacin is used for the prevention of intracranial haemorrhage (Ment et al 1994).

After the first dose of indomethacin transient effects on the quantity of spontaneous movements were described (Bos et al 2000). The incidence and duration of several movement patterns, such as GMs, isolated limb movements and twitches, were substantially reduced, and the incidence and duration of rest periods were increased. The quality of GMs did not change due to indomethacin. However, applying the detailed scoring of GMs as described in Chapter 3 (Fig. 3.8), a reduction in speed was found. Bos et al (2000) recommend a cautious use of bolus indomethacin for the treatment of patent ductus arteriosus.

Until recently, dexamethasone was frequently used in preterm infants at risk for chronic lung disease. However, mortality rates do not decline markedly after postnatal corticosteroid therapy and concern has been raised about its neurological sequelae (Doyle and Davis 2000, Shinwell et al 2000).

In their first study on the effect of dexamethasone therapy Bos and co-workers (1998b) reported on a transient reduction in motility and a reduction of speed and amplitude of GMs during preterm age. In a second study on a much larger sample, particularly with initially normal GMs, the same authors reported changes in the GM quality (Bos et al 2002a). Nine out of 13 infants who initially showed normal GMs developed abnormal GMs immediately after dexamethasone therapy. Two of these infants still had abnormal fidgety movements at 3 months postterm; however it was less certain whether dexamethasone was also to blame for the long-term effects. Chronic lung disease with repeated episodes of hypoxia could also have contributed to the later deficits (Bos et al 2002a).

Systemic diseases do not mimic brain lesion

A serious concern was the question whether a systemic disease, such as infection without brain involvement (candida species, coagulase-negative staphylococcus, staphylococcus aureus), might mimic impairment of GM quality similar to that in brain dysfunction. Bos et al (1997a) could demonstrate that septicaemia has a limited influence on the GM quality. At first sight, GMs can be mistaken for poor repertoire. However, the richness in complexity and variability, in particular of the sequence of the moving body parts, including superimposed rotations, was strictly different from truly poor repertoire GMs. GMs of preterm infants with severe infection just have a sluggish character with a slow speed. Hence, it is possible to discriminate between abnormal GMs due to brain lesion and sluggish GMs due to severe systemic infection, when the complexity of the GMs is considered as the main characteristic for normal GMs (Bos 1993, Bos et al 1997a).

The sluggishness might be explained by changes in muscle function. During septicaemia the resting membrane potential in muscle cells is increased (Cunningham et al 1971, Shiono et al 1989), glucose transport in muscle tissue is impaired (Westfall and Sayeed 1988) and protein breakdown in muscle tissue is enhanced (Hasselgren et al 1988).

Avoiding confusion between abnormal general movements and seizures

For the less experienced observer it might sometimes be difficult to distinguish between abnormal GMs and seizures. GMs with a poor repertoire show a monotonous sequence of the successive movement components that recalls stereotyped movements of subtle seizures. Similarly, some cramped-synchronised GMs may resemble tonic posturing of focal or generalised tonic seizures.

POOR REPERTOIRE GMS AND SUBTLE SEIZURES IN PRETERM AND FULLTERM INFANTS

Subtle seizures encompass a variety of paroxysmal alterations in neonatal behaviour and motor automatisms (i.e. ocular phenomena, oral-buccal-lingual movements, limb movements, autonomic phenomena, apnoeic spells). Volpe (1995, 2000) described peculiar extremity movements, resembling 'boxing', 'hooking', or 'pedalling'. Mizrahi and Kellaway (1987, 1998) described rowing or swimming movements of the arms and pedalling or bicycling movements of the legs as 'progression movements'.

What is peculiar to seizure movements, but certainly not to poor repertoire GMs, is the extreme stereotypy and the ictal character of the clinical phenomena. The sequence of movements does not change during the single seizure or even in successive seizures. Poor repertoire GMs are monotonous in the sequence but are never stereotyped to such a degree as seizures are. Other ictal motor phenomena such as abnormal eye movements, oral-buccal-lingual movements or autonomic phenomena during limb movements are never seen during poor repertoire GMs.

CRAMPED-SYNCHRONISED GMS AND TONIC SEIZURES IN PRETERM AND FULLTERM INFANTS

Focal tonic and especially generalised tonic seizures can be confused with cramped-synchronised GMs. Focal tonic seizures consist of sustained posturing of a limb or asymmetrical posturing of the trunk or neck, most often associated with EEG seizure discharge. Generalised tonic seizures can be observed as tonic extension of both upper and lower extremities (a decerebrate posture is mimicked), as tonic flexion of upper extremities with extension of lower extremities (a decorticate posture is mimicked), as tonic flexion of the four limbs, or asymmetrical posture of the limbs that mimic the asymmetrical tonic neck posture. Again, the stereotypy in addition to other ictal phenomena (e.g. eye movements, oral automatisms, vegetative phenomena) and the loss of consciousness indicate a tonic seizure and not an abnormality of GMs. Cramped-synchronised GMs, however, are not stereotyped despite all limb and trunk muscles contracting and relaxing almost simultaneously.

If clinical observation does not enable a differentiation between seizure and abnormal GMs, an EEG-recording can be helpful, despite the fact that not all motor automatisms, particularly tonic generalised seizures, are consistently accompanied by epileptic discharges in the EEG.

CRAMPED-SYNCHRONISED GMS AND SEIZURES AFTER THE NEONATAL PERIOD

Infants with severe brain damage, such as full-term infants affected by severe hypoxic-ischaemic encephalopathy and preterm infants affected by severe periventricular leuko-malacia or periventricular haemorrhagic infarction, are at high risk for epilepsy. The risk for recurrence of seizure is higher after neonatal seizures and after abnormalities of the neonatal interictal EEG (Volpe 2000). During the first 2 to 5 months postterm age, tonic seizures and tonic spasms of West syndrome may be confused with cramped-synchronised GMs.

It can be difficult to recognise epileptic spasms as they may be subtle in appearance and brief in duration, extremely heterogeneous in appearance (tonic, myoclonic, in flexion, in extension, in adduction), they occur most often in clusters but sometimes as isolated phenomena, and they may be superimposed on an abnormal motility. The typical spasms, with adduction and semi-flexion of the four limbs and with flexion of the head and trunk, may look similar to cramped-synchronised GMs, but are always much more stereotyped and faster in speed.

Infants with West syndrome are usually irritable, show a low threshold to the Moro response, have tremors and jitteriness, suffer from abnormalities of the muscle tone and may in addition have cramped-synchronised GMs. In case of clinical suspicion, a video-EEG-polygraphical recording should be performed. Clinical spasms coincident with EEG paroxysmal features are a confirmation of West syndrome.

Other tonic epileptic seizures, such as those seen in Ohtahara syndrome or in early myoclonic encephalopathy, are easy to recognise and cannot be confused with cramped-synchronised GMs.

Does sensory stimulation interfere with fidgety movements?

Fidgety movements are only present in the awake infant. They can be observed in any position of the infant but they can be observed best if the infant is supine or sitting in a relaxing chair. As mentioned earlier, fidgety movements can hardly be seen when the infant is crying or fussing since all movements then become jerky, even rigid, and speeded up (see Chapters 2 and 3). A different question is to what extent focused attention to various stimuli could interfere with fidgety movements.

A series of experiments has been carried out to investigate the effects of visual, acoustic, social and proprioceptive stimuli on the quality and temporal organisation of fidgety movements (Dibiasi and Einspieler 2002, 2004). None of the stimuli changed the quality of fidgety movements. However, the results differed for temporal organisation.

A red ring did not attract the attention of 12-week-old infants sufficiently and thus did not change the temporal organisation of fidgety movements. By contrast, visually highly interesting features, such as a red puppet with big eyes (Fig. 4.2), may counteract

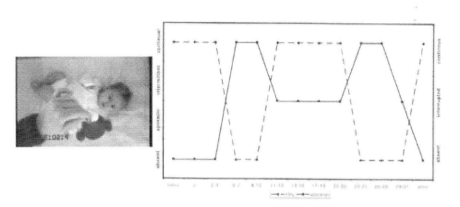

Fig. 4.2 Stimulation with a red puppet (left) causes focused attention counteracting the temporal organisation of fidgety movements (right). During the whole stimulation no fidgety movements were observed (y2-axis, right-hand scale) whereas the infant was continuously looking towards the red puppet (y1-axis, left-hand scale). After the red puppet was removed fidgety movements reappeared in the temporal organisation seen before stimulation (reproduced with permission from Dibiasi and Einspieler 2002).

the temporal organisation of fidgety movements. A decrease or stop of fidgety movements lasted for about 20 seconds and was subsequently followed by an increase.

The practical consequence is that, for the assessment of fidgety movements, interference stemming from highly interesting toys must be avoided. If this is not possible, assessment should be postponed until habituation has taken place and fidgety movements are once again occurring in the expected temporal organisation.

Short and unfamiliar sounds up to 88 dB did not influence the temporal organisation of fidgety movements. It seems unlikely, therefore, that longer-lasting sounds of the same intensity would do so. Consequently, for the application of the GM assessment one need not necessarily assess the infant in a quiet room (Dibiasi and Einspieler 2002).

In contrast to what has been stated previously (Prechtl et al 1997b), fidgety movements are not influenced by social interference. The mother's or experimenter's presence and joyful talking with the infant do not interfere with fidgety movements. Infants may be recorded for the assessment of fidgety movements while the caregiver is in close proximity to the infant or even talking to the infant. A problem that remains is that the analyser's visual Gestalt perception may be impaired if other persons are present during the recording (see Chapter 3).

We consider fidgety movements as an age-specific fine-tuning of the proprioceptive system (Prechtl and Hopkins 1986, Prechtl 2001a). Hence, it was of interest to examine if fidgety movements change during or after proprioceptive stimulation. Bracelets with lead pearls were put on the 3-month-old infant's arms or legs or both, bilaterally and unilaterally. Surprisingly, fidgety movements did not change (Dibiasi and Einspieler 2004). Fidgety movements remained the same even if the infant was weighted on one side with up to 140 grams per arm and leg, respectively (Fig. 4.3).

That various environmental interferences changed neither the quality nor the temporal organisation of fidgety movements once again underlines that the major function of the young nervous system is to generate spontaneous activity: spontaneous activity that is robust and relatively independent of sensory stimulation. Fidgety movements are a transient but very stable and predominant feature of the young nervous system.

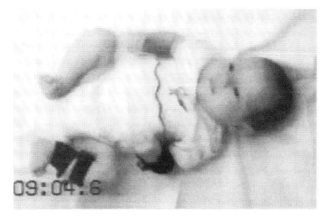

Fig. 4.3 One-sided weighting of the 3-month-old infant with 140 grams on the left arm and the left leg, respectively (Dibiasi and Einspieler 2004).

5

HOW OBJECTIVE, RELIABLE AND VALID IS THE GENERAL MOVEMENT ASSESSMENT?

Inter-observer agreement and test–retest reliability are very high

As the qualitative GM assessment is based on pattern recognition it is of utmost importance that the inter-observer agreement is sufficiently high, and thus the method can be considered as objective. So far, 11 studies on 358 infants assessed by 90 observers have revealed an agreement of between 89 and 93 per cent (Table 5.1). Cohen's kappa is used to assess inter-rater agreement when observing qualitative variables. Kappa is considered to be an improvement over using percentage agreement to evaluate this type of reliability (Cohen 1960). The average kappa in another four studies on 108 infants assessed by 11 observers was 0.88 (Table 5.1).

The effectiveness of training in GM assessment was investigated in 700 participants at various three- to four-day basic training courses. They reached 83 per cent correct

TABLE 5.1
Inter-observer agreement for the assessment of GM quality in 15 studies on a total number of 466 infants. All together 101 observers participated in these studies

	Number of observers	Number of infants observed	Inter-observer agreement (IA) or kappa (K)
Prechtl 1990	10	20	IA = 90%
Van Kranen-Mastenbroek et al 1992	4	30	K = 0.84
Geerdink and Hopkins 1993a	2	35	IA = 87% to 93%
Albers and Jorch 1994	8	22	IA = 67% to 99%
Bos et al 1997a	2	6	IA = 96%
Bos et al 1997b	2	19	K = 0.92
Cioni et al 1997a	2	66	IA = 91%
Cioni et al 1997c	2	58	IA = 87%
Einspieler et al 1997	51	30	IA = 84% to 88%
Bos et al 1998a	2	27	K = 0.84
Bos et al 1998b	2	15	IA = 98%
Cioni et al 2000	3	32	K = 0.91
Bos et al 2000	2	48	IA = 94%
Einspieler et al 2002	2 to 6	36	IA = 92% to 97%
Guzzetta et al 2003	3	22	IA = 92% to 97%

Kappa > 0.75, excellent agreement.

TABLE 5.2
Sensitivity obtained for GM assessment during different age periods in seven different studies

	Preterm period	Writhing movement period	Fidgety movement period	Number of cases	Outcome
Ferrari et al 1990	100%			29 preterms	2 years: cerebral palsy
Geerdink and Hopkins 1993a	60%	80%	100%	35 small-for-gestational-age preterms	1 year: poor outcome according to neurological examination
Prechtl et al 1993		100%	85%	26 full-terms	2 years: cerebral palsy
Cioni et al 1997a	91%	100%	100%	66 preterms	2 years: cerebral palsy and/or developmental retardation
Cioni et al 1997c		94%	94%	58 full-terms	2 years: cerebral palsy and/or developmental retardation
Prechtl et al 1997b			95%	130 pre- and full-terms	2 years: cerebral palsy and/or developmental retardation
Ferrari et al 2002	100%	100%	100%	84 preterms	3 years: cerebral palsy

Developmental retardation = developmental scores more than two standard deviations below normal.

judgements. Additional training of almost 100 participants significantly increased the correct judgements to 89 per cent. If only the global discrimination between normal and abnormal GMs was considered, 94 per cent had correct judgements. Interestingly, it was more difficult to correctly judge infants, if they were recorded around term age (Valentin, personal communication).

An analysis of 20 GM recordings repeated after a time interval of two years obtained a 100 per cent test–retest reliability for global judgement, and an 85 per cent reliability for detailed analysis using the GM optimality list, as described in Chapter 3 (Einspieler 1994).

The validity of the general movement assessment

When introducing an assessment technique the effectiveness must be considered carefully: how accurate is the method when it comes to detecting disease positives, i.e. later neurological deficits; and how accurate is the method at excluding disease negatives, i.e. those who do not have later neurological deficits. The conventional indices employed to determine this are sensitivity and specificity (Bland 1996).

Sensitivity is the number who are both disease positive and test positive divided by the number who are disease positive, in other words the percentage of cases which are correctly identified as high-risk for later neurological impairment (Bland 1996). Table 5.2 provides the details of several studies on GM assessment and the calculated sensitivity values. An overall sensitivity of 94 per cent indicates that only 6 per cent were false negatives. The only exception is the study on GM assessment during preterm age by Geerdink and Hopkins (1993a) with a sensitivity of 60 per cent (Table 5.2). However, this study is not comparable with the others because the outcome was measured at 1 year of age and 'disease positive' was defined as 'poor outcome according to neurological examination'. In all other studies the outcome was measured at the end of the second year, or later, and cerebral palsy or developmental retardation (developmental scores below two standard deviations) or both were taken as 'disease positives'.

Specificity is the number who are both disease negative and test negative divided by the number who are disease negative, in other words the percentage of cases which are correctly identified as normal (Bland 1996). Table 5.3 provides the details of several studies on GM assessment and the calculated specificity values. Specificity was lower during the preterm and writhing movement period (46 to 93 per cent). This was due to the number of infants with abnormal GMs (mainly poor repertoire) at this early age who normalised before or at the fidgety movement period and who had a normal outcome (Fig. 5.1). Thus, with increasing age, specificity increased, revealing values between 82 and 100 per cent during the third month when normal fidgety movements predict a normal neurological outcome.

The largest study so far, in which 130 infants participated, clearly emphasised the importance of the fidgety movements (Prechtl et al 1997b). According to brain ultrasound findings 60 infants were at low risk and 70 at high risk. Ninety-six per cent of the infants with normal fidgety movements had a normal neurological outcome, whereas abnormal quality or total absence of fidgety movements was followed by neurological abnormalities in 95 per cent of the cases (cerebral palsy in 82 per cent and developmental

TABLE 5.3
Specificity obtained for GM assessment during different age periods in seven different studies

	Preterm period	Writhing movement period	Fidgety movement period	Number of cases	Outcome
Ferrari et al 1990	59%			29 preterms	2 years: cerebral palsy
Geerdink and Hopkins 1993a	58%	67%	100%	35 small-for-gestational-age preterms	1 year: poor outcome according to neurological examination
Prechtl et al 1993		46%	82%	26 full-terms	2 years: cerebral palsy
Cioni et al 1997a	58%	70%	85%	66 preterms	2 years: cerebral palsy and/or developmental retardation
Cioni et al 1997c		71%	83%	58 full-terms	2 years: cerebral palsy and/or developmental retardation
Prechtl et al 1997b			96%	130 pre- and full-terms	2 years: cerebral palsy and/or developmental retardation
Ferrari et al 2002	93%	93%	100%	84 preterms	3 years: cerebral palsy

Developmental retardation = developmental scores more than two standard deviations below normal.

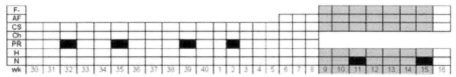

retardation and minor neurological signs in 13 per cent). Several other studies confirmed

Fig. 5.1 Individual developmental trajectory of case 1 born at 30 weeks postmenstrual age. Poor repertoire GMs during preterm and term age are followed by normal fidgety movements. Outcome (4 years): normal.

F-, absence of fidgety movements; AF, abnormal fidgety movements; CS, cramped-synchronised GMs; Ch, chaotic GMs; PR, poor repertoire GMs; H, hypokinesis; N, normal GMs; wk, weeks. The age period where fidgety movements are obligatory is marked in grey.

the high correlation between fidgety movements and neurological outcome (Bos et al 1997b, 1998b, Cioni et al 2000, Einspieler et al 2002, Ferrari et al 2002, Guzzetta et al 2003).

The likelihood ratios (LR) are dependent on sensitivity and specificity. They indicate a figure by which a positive (LR+) or a negative test result (LR-) changes the odds for really having the disease. The higher the LR+ and the lower the LR-, the better a test is. In general, an LR+ > 10 and an LR- < 0.1 characterises a very good test (Sackett et al 2000).

Calculating the LRs from previous results (Prechtl et al 1997b) gives an LR+ for cramped-synchronised GMs of 45 (95 per cent confidence interval: 6.4 to 321), and an LR+ for poor repertoire GMs of only 0.61 (95 per cent confidence interval: 0.40 to 0.93). For normal preterm and writhing GMs the LR- is 0.04 (95 per cent confidence interval: 0.005 to 0.27). The LR+ for an absence of fidgety movements is > 51, and for abnormal fidgety movements it is 5.1 (95 per cent confidence interval: 1.5 to 17), whereas the LR- for normal fidgety movements is 0.05 (95 per cent confidence interval: 0.02 to 0.17). Thus, normal GMs at any age as well as cramped-synchronised GMs and the absence of fidgety movements have excellent LRs.

Specific signs predicting cerebral palsy

The traditional approach to diagnosing cerebral palsy is to detect the first signs of this neurological condition at the age of 8 to 12 months postterm. At this age, the first signs of spasticity, or pareses, or merely of consistent hypertonia, or any other signs specific for one or other form of cerebral palsy, may be detected. Perlman (1998) stated that no early markers for the later development of cerebral palsy are recognisable in the neonatal period, but he was referring to the traditional neurological examination.

The change in paradigm from the traditional testing of reflexes, responses and tonus to a new assessment technique, which focuses on the quality of GMs, is indeed a diagnostic breakthrough (see Chapter 1). With the qualitative assessment of GMs, it is now possible to detect prenatally in the foetus, or postnatally in the preterm or term infant, specific neurological signs which are highly predictive for the later development of cerebral palsy.

CONSISTENT CRAMPED-SYNCHRONISED GENERAL MOVEMENTS AND THE
ABSENCE OF FIDGETY MOVEMENTS PREDICT SPASTIC CEREBRAL PALSY

The first longitudinal study on the predictive value of the various abnormal GM patterns revealed cramped-synchronised GMs (for a definition see Chapter 2) as highly predictive for a severe neurological outcome (Ferrari et al 1990). The largest longitudinal study of 130 infants, consisting of the whole spectrum of brain ultrasound findings due to hypoxic-ischaemic lesions or haemorrhages, confirmed the importance of cramped-synchronised GMs. All children who at repeated examinations showed consistently cramped-synchronised GMs (N = 40) later developed severe spastic cerebral palsy (Fig. 5.2; Prechtl et al 1997b).

In a recent study of 84 preterm infants with brain lesion indicated by ultrasound scan, Ferrari et al (2002) reported that the earlier consistent cramped-synchronised GMs occur, the worse the later motor impairment. The severity was scored at the age of at least 3 years in accordance with a system of classification of gross motor functions in children with cerebral palsy (Palisano et al 1997).

Exceptionally, less dramatic signs, such as the consistent presence of poor repertoire GMs, may also lead to cerebral palsy (Fig. 5.2; Prechtl et al 1997b). This observation suggests that a poor repertoire of GMs should not merely be considered as a mild abnormality, as has been recently suggested (Hadders-Algra et al 1997).

So far, we have never seen consistently normal GMs followed by cerebral palsy, provided there were no severe interval complications. Thus, we had no cases of false negative findings (Fig. 5.2).

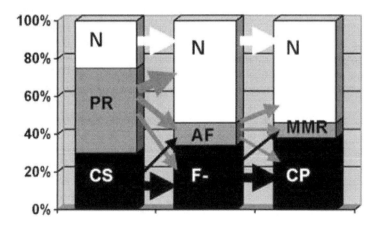

Fig. 5.2 A longitudinal study on 130 infants with various ultrasound findings: writhing movement quality (left) preceding the quality of fidgety movements (middle), which is predictive for the neurological outcome at 2 to 3 years (right) (Prechtl et al 1997b).

N, normal (writhing movements, fidgety movements, outcome); PR, poor repertoire GMs; CS, cramped-synchronised GMs; AF, abnormal fidgety movements; F-, absence of fidgety movements; MMR, mental or motor retardation or both; CP, cerebral palsy.

Consistent findings refer to about bi-weekly recordings during the preterm period, one recording during the term period, and at least one additional recording during the first two months postterm.

There is yet another early marker for later development of cerebral palsy. In the study mentioned above (Prechtl et al 1997b), only three out of 70 infants with normal fidgety movements had later cognitive or motor impairment or both, and 67 (96 per cent) were normal at 2 years of age; none developed cerebral palsy (Fig. 5.2). On the other hand, 44 out of 130 infants never showed fidgety movements and 43 of them (98 per cent) developed severe spastic cerebral palsy. The remaining infant, who had a poor repertoire of GMs in his pre-fidgety movement period, had severe cognitive and motor impairment. Less clear are the prognoses of those infants who showed the exaggerated type of abnormal fidgety movements (N = 16 out of 130). Three cases turned out normal, seven became cognitively or motorically impaired, and six (37 per cent) developed cerebral palsy (Fig. 5.2). However, all six cases with cerebral palsy had consistently cramped-synchronised GMs before showing abnormal fidgety movements. In addition, it is remarkable that of the seven cases that had consistently poor repertoire GMs during their first weeks of life but later developed cerebral palsy, none had ever developed fidgety movements.

Thus, in addition to consistently cramped-synchronised GMs during preterm and early postterm age, the absence of fidgety movements is a specific sign of later spastic cerebral palsy.

In conclusion, specific early signs of later spastic cerebral palsy are consistently cramped-synchronised GMs (Fig. 5.3) or absence of fidgety movements (Fig. 5.4) or both (Fig. 5.5). Both abnormal qualities of GMs can be seen at an age at which no clinical evidence of cerebral palsy is yet present, namely as early as from foetal life onwards or from preterm or term birth until the third month postterm (Prechtl et al 1997b).

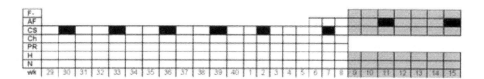

Fig. 5.3 Individual developmental trajectory of case 2 born at 28 weeks postmenstrual age. Consistent cramped-synchronised GMs during the preterm, term and early postterm period are followed by abnormal fidgety movements. Outcome: spastic cerebral palsy. Abbreviations as in Fig. 5.1.

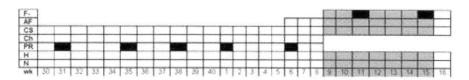

Fig. 5.4 Individual developmental trajectory of case 3 born at 29 weeks postmenstrual age. Consistent poor repertoire GMs during the preterm, term and early postterm period are followed by absence of fidgety movements. Outcome: spastic cerebral palsy. Abbreviations as in Fig. 5.1.

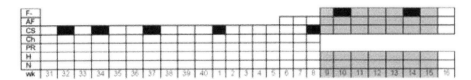

Fig. 5.5 Individual developmental trajectory of case 4 born at 30 weeks postmenstrual age. Consistent cramped-synchronised GMs during the preterm, term and early postterm period are followed by an absence of fidgety movements. Outcome: spastic cerebral palsy. Abbreviations as in Fig. 5.1.

The validity of normal fidgety movements on the one hand, and the absence of fidgety movements on the other hand, is clearly demonstrated if we deal with an individual developmental trajectory with transient cramped-synchronised GMs. Transient cramped-synchronised GMs may lead to cerebral palsy if fidgety movements are absent (Fig. 5.6). If transient cramped-synchronised GMs are followed by normal fidgety movements, the neurological outcome may be normal (Fig. 5.7; Ferrari et al 2002).

EARLY DIFFERENTIAL SIGNS OF LATER SPASTIC DIPLEGIA VERSUS TETRAPLEGIA
Consistent cramped-synchronised GMs predict both spastic diplegia and tetraplegia. Cases with later diplegia have a later onset and shorter duration of cramped-synchronised GMs than cases with later tetraplegia (Ferrari et al 2002). If, in addition to the cramped-synchronised GMs, so-called segmental movements are frequently present in the upper limbs, the child will most probably develop diplegia (Cioni et al 1997b). Segmental movements are distinct movements of hand and feet, fingers and toes, occurring either

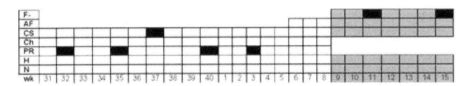

Fig. 5.6 Individual developmental trajectory of case 5 born at 30 weeks postmenstrual age. Poor repertoire GMs during preterm, term and early postterm period; cramped-synchronised GMs at 37 weeks; absence of fidgety movements. Outcome: spastic cerebral palsy. Abbreviations as in Fig. 5.1.

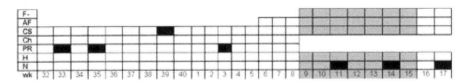

Fig. 5.7 Individual developmental trajectory of case 6 born at 31 weeks postmenstrual age. Poor repertoire GMs during preterm, term and early postterm period; cramped-synchronised GMs at 39 weeks; normal fidgety movements. Outcome (3 years): normal. Abbreviations as in Fig. 5.1.

isolated or as part of GMs. In the latter case they are not part of limb flexion or extension (Cioni et al 1997b, van der Heide et al 1999, Cioni et al 2000).

EARLY SIGNS OF HEMIPLEGIA
Often, congenital hemiplegia, the most frequent type of cerebral palsy in term infants, and the second most frequent in preterm infants after diplegia, is only diagnosed after the first year of life. Whether this late diagnosis is due to a delayed onset of the clinical signs, or to an initial neglect of neurological signs already present, remains unclear.

From neonatal age onwards, neuroimaging techniques provide the possibility of identifying brain lesions, mainly cerebral infarctions, which may cause hemiplegia. Consequently, it is now possible to perform prospective studies on the neurological development of these infants. In order to investigate whether the assessment of GMs may help in the earlier detection of hemiplegia, two different studies were carried out: the first on 16 preterm infants with unilateral intraparenchymal echodensity at brain ultrasound, most likely venous infarctions (Cioni et al 2000); and the second on 11 term infants with cerebral infarction on brain magnetic resonance imaging (Guzzetta et al 2003). All infants with subsequent hemiplegia had an absence of fidgety movements following bilateral cramped-synchronised or poor repertoire GMs. The observation of abnormal movements from birth onwards refutes the hypothesis of a silent period of later hemiplegia.

The first asymmetric sign, independent of the head position, is segmental movements (as described above), which are reduced or absent contra-lateral to the side of the lesion (Cioni et al 2000, Guzzetta et al 2003). This asymmetry occurs in preterm-born infants from 3 months postterm age onwards (Cioni et al 2000). In term-born infants with neonatal infarction the asymmetry of segmental movements is already present during the second month (Guzzetta et al 2003).

EARLY SIGNS OF LATER DYSKINETIC CEREBRAL PALSY
Recently, it has also been possible to document early markers specifically predictive for the development of dyskinetic cerebral palsy. A dyskinetic group of 12 cases (Einspieler et al 2002) comprised syndromes of choreo-athethosis as well as dystonic forms (Hagberg and Hagberg 1993).

Until the second month postterm, the infant who will later become dyskinetic displays a poor repertoire of GMs, 'arm movements in circles' and finger spreading. Characteristically, these abnormal arm and finger movements remain until at least 5 months postterm. The abnormal unilateral or bilateral 'arm movements in circles' should not be confused with normal writhing or swiping arm movements. The normal writhing character of GMs consists of ellipsoid arm movements of variable speed, intensity and amplitude, while swiping arm movements are ballistic, fast, of large amplitude and high speed (see Chapter 2). In contrast to these normal movements, the abnormal 'arm movements in circles' are monotonous, slow, forward rotations from the shoulder. The monotony in speed and amplitude, in particular, is the most characteristic quality of 'arm movements in circles'. Usually these abnormal arm movements are accompanied by finger spreading (Einspieler et al 2002).

A lack of movements towards the midline, particularly foot–foot contact, is an additional specific sign of later dyskinetic cases. In addition, the majority of cases displayed neither hand–hand contact nor hand–mouth contact.

By contrast, as reported earlier (Illingworth 1966, Bobath 1971, Vining et al 1976, Taft 1995), an obligatory asymmetric tonic neck response before the sixth month did not discriminate between infants who developed normally and those who developed either spastic or dyskinetic cerebral palsy (Einspieler et al 2002).

Common to both spastic and dyskinetic cases was the absence of fidgety movements and the absence of antigravity movements, i.e. legs lifting, during the third to fifth month. The absence of fidgety movements is of particular interest. Prechtl (1997a) suggested a specific central pattern generator for fidgety movements, located, most likely, in the brainstem (see Chapter 2). The absence of fidgety movements in both forms of cerebral palsy, caused by different brain lesions, indicates that intact cortico-spinal fibres as well as the output from the basal ganglia and cerebellum are necessary to generate normal fidgety movements (Einspieler et al 2002).

Prediction of neurological deficits other than cerebral palsy
Abnormal fidgety movements (see Chapter 2) are less predictive for the neurological outcome than the absence of fidgety movements (Prechtl et al 1997b) but have been discussed in the context of the development of mild neurological deficits, by at least 2 to 3 years of age (Bos et al 1997b, 1999, 2002b, Zavrl, personal communication). In addition to the abnormal quality of fidgety movements, Bos et al (2002b) pointed out that a monotonous character of the repertoire of other movements increased the probability of the development of mild neurological deficits, such as tonus abnormalities, co-ordination problems and gross motor problems. In the group of infants with mild deficits at 2 years, the occurrence of movements towards the midline, mutual hand contact, manipulation and fiddling movements (for a description of these patterns, see Chapter 2) emerged on average two to three weeks later than in the normal infants. However, this finding did not have predictive value for the individual infant.

A study on some 50 children indicated that mildly abnormal GMs at 3 to 4 months (fidgety movement period) have a prognostic significance, pointing to an increased risk for the development of minor neurological deficits, attention deficit hyperactivity disorder, and boisterous, disobedient behaviour in 4- to 9-year-old children (Hadders-Algra and Groothuis 1999). However, their definition of 'mildly abnormal GMs' during the fidgety movement period differs greatly from Prechtl's GM assessment (see Chapter 10). According to Hadders-Algra et al (1997), mildly abnormal GMs lack the fluency but still show some complexity and variation.

In the context of a study on possible long-term effects of infantile apnoeas, we were able to evaluate the long-term prediction of fidgety movements. The participants were 33 girls and boys, now 11 to 15 years old. Children with a history of abnormal fidgety movements had lower Griffiths scores (Brandt 1983) at 2 years (p < 0.05) and lower scores in the Bruininks Oseretsky Test (Bruininks 1978), particularly in fine motor performance (p < 0.01), during mid-puberty. The findings of the neurological examination during pre- and mid-puberty (Touwen 1979) were not related to the GM quality.

Fidgety movements (between 12 and 16 weeks postterm age) with an intermittent temporal organisation (for a definition, see Chapter 2) might be more often related to later mild neurological dysfunction than continuous fidgety movements (Bos, Einspieler and Milioti, personal communication).

After Prechtl had discovered the existence of fidgety movements as an age-specific distinct form of GMs, he speculated about the possible biological function of this transient movement pattern (Prechtl and Hopkins 1986, Prechtl 1997a; see Chapter 2). A possible ontogenetic adaptive function of these ongoing small movements could be conjectured in a re-calibration of the proprioceptive system. This is supported by the fact that fidgety movements occur at the three-month major transformation of many neural functions (Prechtl 1986) and precede visual hand regard and the onset of intentional reaching and visually controlled manipulation of objects. As many aspects of the adaptation to the extra-uterine condition are not reached before the third month of postterm age – the proprioceptive system is still tuned to the intra-uterine condition – a re-calibration of this sensory system could be mandatory for providing the proper control of later fine motor activity. The findings in blind infants (see Chapter 6), as well as the fine motor disability in children with a history of abnormal fidgety movements, support this conjecture.

6
THE CLINICAL APPLICATION OF THE METHOD

A heterogeneous series of clinical conditions such as periventricular leukomalacia, intra-cranial haemorrhages, hypoxic-ischaemic encephalopathy, chronic lung disease, infantile apnoeas, brain malformations and spina bifida aperta, Rett syndrome, intra-uterine growth retardation, maternal diabetes, and early blindness affects the quality of GMs. This chapter provides case histories including individual developmental trajectories and the child's neurological outcome.

Periventricular leukomalacia (PVL) and flares

Lesions in the periventricular white matter, especially if they evolve into extensive cystic lesions, are predictive of later severe motor deficits (Fazzi et al 1994). They affect the quality of GMs. Poor repertoire or cramped-synchronised GMs if followed by the absence of fidgety movements are clearly related to an unfavourable outcome.

Much more common are echodensities in the periventricular white matter, also called 'flares', which do not lead to cysts or ventricular dilatation. MRI investigations have revealed that up to 50 to 75 per cent of preterm infants, most with apparently normal outcomes, may have diffuse white matter lesions (Counsell et al 2003). Therefore, the significance of periventricular echodensities on ultrasound is unclear. GM assessment could help in elucidating this problem as there is a clear relationship between the presence, duration and localisation of transient periventricular echodensities and the developmental course of the GM quality (Ferrari et al 1990, Bos et al 1998a).

Transient periventricular echodensities, particularly in the parieto-occipital white matter, persisting beyond 14 days are related to individual developmental trajectories of abnormal GMs (Fig. 6.1; Bos et al 1998a).

Echodensities with a duration of up to 14 days may result in either abnormal (Fig. 6.2) or normal individual developmental trajectories (Fig. 6.3, Bos et al 1998a). This can be explained by the diverse conditions causing the increased echogenicity, such as venous congestion (Baarsma et al 1987, de Vries LS et al 1992), oedema (de Vries LS et al 1988), microscopic haemorrhage (DiPietro et al 1986), necrosis, microcysts and gliosis (Leviton and Paneth 1990).

Echodensities in the frontal white matter which resolve before the fourteenth day of life do not have any impact on the GM quality (Bos et al 1998a). This is in accordance with reports on favourable outcome after isolated frontal cerebral lesion (Fazzi et al 1994, Rademaker et al 1994).

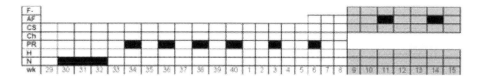

Fig. 6.1 Individual developmental trajectory of case 7 born at 29 weeks postmenstrual age. Brain ultrasound: transient periventricular echodensity in the parieto-occipital white matter (5 weeks). Normal GMs are followed by poor repertoire GMs and abnormal fidgety movements. Outcome (24 months): fine motor abilities impaired (Bos et al 1998a).

F-, absence of fidgety movements; AF, abnormal fidgety movements; CS, cramped-synchronised GMs; Ch, chaotic GMs; PR, poor repertoire GMs; H, hypokinesis; N, normal GMs; wk, weeks. The age period where fidgety movements are obligatory is marked in grey.

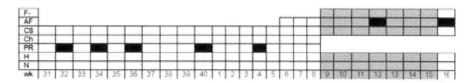

Fig. 6.2 Individual developmental trajectory of case 8 born at 30 weeks postmenstrual age. Brain ultrasound: transient periventricular echodensity in the parieto-occipital white matter until the sixth day. Poor repertoire GMs and abnormal fidgety movements. Outcome (24 months): hypertonia and poor coordination (Bos et al 1998a). Abbreviations as in Fig. 6.1.

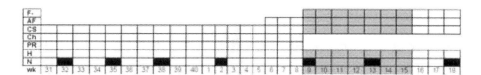

Fig. 6.3 Individual developmental trajectory of case 9 born at 30 weeks postmenstrual age. Brain ultrasound: transient periventricular echodensity in the parieto-occipital white matter until the sixth day. GMH-IVH (germinal matrix intraventricular haemorrhage) grade 1 (Volpe 1989) left. Normal writhing movements followed by normal fidgety movements. Outcome (24 months): normal (Bos et al 1998a). Abbreviations as in Fig. 6.1.

Intracranial haemorrhage

Infants with moderate (grade 2, Volpe 1989) and severe (grade 3 and 3 plus, Volpe 1989) intracranial haemorrhages may consistently have GMs of abnormal quality. These qualitative abnormalities are related to an abnormal neurological outcome (Fig. 6.4; Ferrari et al 1990).

Infants with GMH-IVH grade 1 (Volpe 1989) may develop neurologically abnormally or may have a normal outcome. In such cases the qualitative assessment of GMs is of great help. Infants with consistently abnormal GMs will develop neurological deficits (Fig. 6.5), whereas a normalisation of GMs, particularly normal fidgety movements, predicts a normal neurological outcome (Fig. 6.6).

47

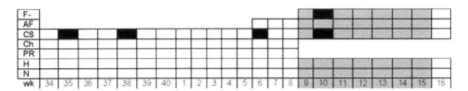

Fig. 6.4 Individual developmental trajectory of case 10 born at 33 weeks postmenstrual age (twin pregnancy). Brain ultrasound at 33 weeks: GMH-IVH grade 1 (Volpe 1989) and ventricular asymmetry (left > right); at 34 weeks: GMH-IVH grade 3 (left > right), diffuse periventricular increased echogenicity, ventricular dilatation (left > right); at 35 weeks: reduced haemorrhage, bilateral multiple cysts, ventricular dilatation (left > right); at 39 weeks: ditto. MRI (magnetic resonance imaging) at 8 months postterm: diffuse periventricular and subcortical increased signal at protonic density and T2, ventricular diffuse dilatation, dilatation of subarachnoidal space, cortical atrophy. Cramped-synchronised GMs and absence of fidgety movements. Outcome (22 months): spastic tetraplegia, learning disability, visual cortical deficit (Ferrari et al 1990). Abbreviations as in Fig. 6.1.

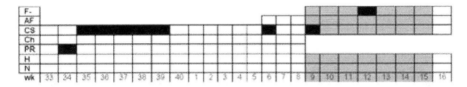

Fig. 6.5 Individual developmental trajectory of case 11 born at 32 weeks postmenstrual age. Brain ultra-sound at 34 weeks: GMH-IVH grade 1 (Volpe 1989); prolonged periventricular increased echogenicity. Poor repertoire followed by consistent cramped-synchronised GMs and absence of fidgety movements. Outcome (18 months): spastic diplegia, no learning disability, DQ (developmental quotient) (Brunet and Lezine 1967) = 90, strabismus (Ferrari et al 1990). Abbreviations as in Fig. 6.1.

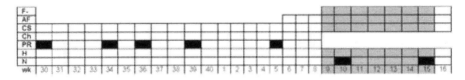

Fig. 6.6 Individual developmental trajectory of case 12 born at 27.3 weeks postmenstrual age. Brain ultrasound at 27.4 and 28 weeks: frontal increased echogenicity; 29 weeks: ditto and right GMH-IVH grade 2 (Volpe 1989); 31 weeks: frontal and occipital increased echogenicity, right GMH-IVH grade 2; 39 weeks: small right frontal cyst. Poor repertoire GMs and normal fidgety movements. Outcome (18 months): no abnormal signs, DQ = 98 (Griffiths 1954, Ferrari et al 1990). Abbreviations as in Fig. 6.1.

Unilateral lesions

Preterm infants with a unilateral increased parenchymal echodensity, very likely as a result of a venous infarction, have a high risk for hemiplegia. GM assessment helps to identify those infants who will later develop hemiplegia (Fig. 6.7) and those who will not (Fig. 6.8). The early signs of hemiplegia are described in detail in Chapter 5. Cramped-synchronised

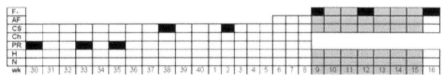

GMs and an absence of fidgety movements (both abnormalities are bilateral) as well as a
Fig. 6.7 Individual developmental trajectory of case 13 born at 26 weeks postmenstrual age. Brain ultrasound: left increased periventricular echodensity, frontal and parietal. Neurological examination: (Dubowitz and Dubowitz 1981) normal findings during the preterm period; (Prechtl 1977) hypertonia, hyperexcitability and asymmetry during term age; hypertonia and asymmetries during the third month. The movement asymmetry score (Cioni et al 2000) revealed no asymmetries during the preterm period, more age-adequate movements on the left side from term age onwards and more segmental movements on the left side from the third month onwards. Poor repertoire followed by cramped-synchronised GMs, absence of fidgety movements. Outcome (24 months): right hemiplegia (Cioni et al 2000). Abbreviations as in Fig. 6.1.

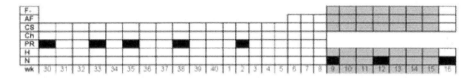

Fig. 6.8 Individual developmental trajectory of case 14 born at 26 weeks postmenstrual age. Brain ultrasound: left increased periventricular echodensity, frontal. Neurological examination: (Dubowitz and Dubowitz 1981) hypotonia during the preterm period; (Prechtl 1977) hypotonia and hyperexcitability during term age; normal findings at 3 months. The movement asymmetry score (Cioni et al 2000) revealed no asymmetries. More segmental movements on the left side from the third month onwards. Poor repertoire GMs and normal fidgety movements. Outcome (24 months): normal (Cioni et al 2000). Abbreviations as in Fig. 6.1.

reduction of segmental movements on the side contra-lateral to the lesion (from 3 months onwards) are highly predictive for hemiplegia (Cioni et al 2000).

Cerebral infarction in term infants is not always followed by later neuromotor sequelae (Wulfeck et al 1991, de Vries LS et al 1997, Estan and Hope 1997, Guzzetta et al 2003). Whereas GM abnormalities during the early postterm period do not always differentiate between later hemiplegia and normal outcome, the fidgety movements are highly predictive (Guzzetta et al 2003). Figs 6.9 and 6.10 demonstrate two similar case histories: abnormal GMs predicting hemiplegia (Fig. 6.9); and normal GMs predicting a normal motor outcome (Fig. 6.10).

In contrast to preterm infants with focal lesions who later develop hemiplegia, term infants have an earlier onset of the asymmetry of segmental movements, at 3 to 6 weeks. This difference is probably due to the timing and type of lesion. In preterm newborns the lesion occurs at an earlier stage of brain development when neurological functions are perhaps less clearly localised, and the pattern of lesion is different. Even when these preterm infants show a predominantly unilateral lesion they also have contra-lateral densities or

49

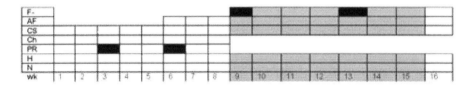

Fig. 6.9 Individual developmental trajectory of case 15 born at term age. Brain ultrasound and MRI (at the seventh day): infarction of a left cortical branch of the medial cerebral artery. The lesion involved the parietal and temporal lobe, the basal ganglia and the internal capsule. More segmental movements on the left side at 3 to 6 weeks, but no asymmetry at 9 to 16 weeks. Poor repertoire GMs and absence of fidgety movements. Outcome (24 months): right hemiplegia (Guzzetta et al 2003). Abbreviations as in Fig. 6.1.

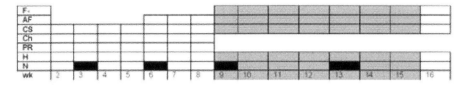

Fig. 6.10 Individual developmental trajectory of case 16 born at term age. Brain ultrasound and MRI (at the fifth day): infarction of a left cortical branch of the medial cerebral artery. More segmental movements on the left side at 3 to 6 weeks, but no asymmetry at 9 to 16 weeks. Normal writhing movements and normal fidgety movements. Outcome (24 months): normal (Guzzetta et al 2003). Abbreviations as in Fig. 6.1.

ventricular dilatation, which may explain the long-lasting presence of transient bilateral neurological signs. In contrast, arterial territory infarction in the term infant is less frequently accompanied by contra-lateral tissue involvement (Guzzetta et al 2003).

Hypoxic ischaemic encephalopathy (HIE) in fullterm infants

In the first days of life most asphyxiated infants show a generalised reduction of motility (hypokinesis – for a definition see Chapter 3). As soon as the infant starts moving, GMs are usually abnormal and tremulous. The degree of hypoxic ischaemic encephalopathy (HIE) according to Sarnat and Sarnat (1976) strongly correlates with the severity and duration of the abnormal changes of the GMs (Prechtl et al 1993). In this respect, the results of neuroimaging correlate with GM abnormalities (Fig. 6.11). However, there are infants with abnormal GMs, particularly in the first two weeks, and normal brain ultrasound findings (Fig. 6.12). Moreover, there are infants with documented morphological changes and transient changes in GMs. If GMs normalised, the outcome was favourable (Fig. 6.13).

Chronic lung disease

Very low birth weight infants at risk for chronic lung disease are also at risk for brain abnormalities such as increased echogenicity, leukomalacia, and intracranial haemorrhage. Therefore, preterm infants with bronchopulmonary dysplasia (BPD) have a worse neuro-developmental outcome than preterms without BPD (Bregman and Farrell 1992).

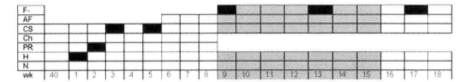

Fig. 6.11 Individual developmental trajectory of case 17 born at 40 weeks; late foetal heart rate decelerations; outborn; Apgar 2 at 5 minutes, intubated; transfer to neonatal intensive care unit at 3 hours; hyperexcitability syndrome (Prechtl 1977), neonatal status epilepticus (until tenth day). Brain ultrasound at 2 days: diffuse white matter and basal ganglia increased echogenicity; at 1 week: ditto and thalamic echogenicity; at 2 weeks: ditto; at 3 weeks: ditto, subcortical cysts, enlarged subarachnoidal spaces, moderate ventricular dilatation. MRI at 4 weeks: moderate ventricular dilatation, enlarged subarachnoidal spaces, diffuse periventricular, subcortical, and basal ganglia increased signal at protonic density and T2 (cortical and subcortical atrophy). Hypokinesis followed by poor repertoire and cramped-synchronised GMs; fast tremulous movements from 2 to 5 weeks; absence of fidgety movements. Outcome (24 months): tetraplegia, epilepsy, severe learning disability (untestable), head circumference < 3rd percentile (Prechtl et al 1993). Abbreviations as in Fig. 6.1.

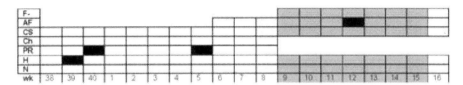

Fig. 6.12 Individual developmental trajectory of case 18 born at 39 weeks; late foetal heart rate decelerations, meconium aspiration, Apgar 3 at 5 minutes, intubated, tracheal suction, hyperexcitability syndrome for three days (Prechtl 1977), moderate EEG abnormalities. Repeated brain ultrasound scans were normal. Hypokinesis followed by poor repertoire and abnormal fidgety movements. Outcome (24 months): motor and cognitive retardation, autistic behaviour, DQ (Griffiths 1954) <50 (Prechtl et al 1993). Abbreviations as in Fig. 6.1.

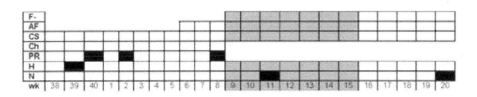

Fig. 6.13 Individual developmental trajectory of case 19 born at 39 weeks; late foetal heart rate decelerations, cord prolapse, stained and slimy amniotic fluid; outborn; Apgar 5 at 5 minutes, resuscitation bag and mask, transferred to neonatal intensive care unit at 6 hours, neonatal status epilepticus until 4 days. Brain ultrasound at 2 days: reduced ventricular size, diffuse periventricular increased echogenicity, mild increased thalamic echogenicity; at 1 week: diffuse white matter increased echogenicity (left > right), more pronounced in frontal and occipital lobes; at 3 weeks: enlarged subarachnoidal spaces, dyshomogeneous increased white matter echogenicity. MRI at 5 weeks: diffuse increased signal (at protonic density and T2) of hemispheric white matter and basal ganglia. Moderate ventricular dilatation, enlarged subarachnoidal spaces (cortical and subcortical atrophy). Hypokinesis followed by poor repertoire and normal fidgety movements. Outcome (17 months): no abnormal signs; DQ (Griffiths 1954) = 98 (Prechtl et al 1993). Abbreviations as in Fig. 6.1.

51

A case report on an infant with severe BPD provided a detailed description of a spontaneous movement disorder at 2 to 3 months postterm called 'infantile chorea', because the movement characteristics and EMG bursting pattern resemble those of adult chorea. The authors assumed a dysfunction of the striato-thalamic circuitry (Hadders-Algra et al 1994).

Dexamethasone treatment is frequently used in infants with BPD to facilitate weaning from the ventilator (Cummings et al 1989). If dexamethasone treatment is required, both the GM quantity and the quality will be transiently affected (Bos et al 1998a, 2002a). Chapter 4 provides details about the effect of dexamethasone on GMs. The improvement of respiratory symptoms, as measured by the number of days on the ventilator after initiating dexamethasone treatment, is not associated with the change in the GM quality (Bos et al 2002a).

In some infants GM abnormalities persist until 3 months postterm and even beyond. The question of whether dexamethasone therapy is to blame for fidgety movement abnormalities remains open. Repeated episodes of hypoxia might also contribute to these findings. Fidgety movements – their presence or absence as well as their normal or abnormal quality – again are highly predictive for the outcome (Bos et al 2002a).

Despite the impairment of GMs after dexamethasone was initiated, no significant increase of brain damage was found on ultrasound scans. Those infants whose brain ultrasound scans indicated worsening of brain damage already had abnormal GMs before dexamethasone treatment commenced (Bos et al 2002a). The authors discussed this finding in line with animal research showing that corticosteroids given before hypoxia reduce hypoxia-induced brain damage, but when administered after the actual insult, aggravate the lesion (Tuor et al 1993, Tsubota et al 1999).

Infantile apnoeas

An apparent life-threatening event (ALTE) in infants is mainly reported by caregivers as a frightening episode. They describe their infant as suddenly becoming apnoeic, pale or cyanotic, and limp. Vigorous stimulation and even cardiopulmonary resuscitation is needed. This is a heterogeneous group of infants, many of whom appear normal following the ALTE. There are many possible diagnoses, but they correlate poorly with the presenting symptoms (Gray et al 1999, Farrell et al 2002).

In addition to polysomnographic and metabolic studies, the neurological development of these infants was the focus of interest. The reported reduction of movements during sleep (Coons and Guilleminault 1985, Schechtman et al 1992) was partially replicated in a detailed observational study. The rate of GMs during sleep only decreased a few months after the ALTE (Einspieler et al 1994).

The frequently observed tremulous GMs after the ALTE are in accordance with the observations in asphyxiated newborns (Prechtl et al 1993). Tremulous writhing movements were noted for a prolonged period during sleep (Einspieler et al 1994), but also during wakefulness (Einspieler 1994). In addition, symmetrical arm movements, sometimes of slow speed, prolonged full extension of fingers followed by slow closure, or head banging during sleep were observed (Einspieler et al 1994). Cramped-synchronised GMs were

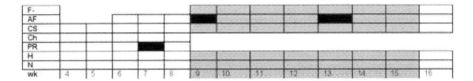

Fig. 6.14 Individual developmental trajectory of case 20 born at term; apparent life-threatening event at 5 weeks, detailed clinical examination revealed no cause. Poor repertoire but tremulous GMs, abnormal fidgety movements. Outcome (14 years): minor neurological dysfunction according to Touwen (1979), fine manipulative disabilities, poor quality of movements, dyskinesia, poor co-ordination of extremities; low score in the Bruininks Oseretsky Test (Bruininks 1978). Abbreviations as in Fig. 6.1.

present in only one out of 21 infants with ALTE. This child developed severe cognitive and moderate motor retardation (outcome at 15 years of age). Abnormal fidgety movements were rare but indicative for later fine motor disabilities. Fig. 6.14 illustrates a case history.

In the context of research and prevention of sudden infant death the analysis of respiratory patterns and apnoeas has received perhaps undue attention. However, the relationship between repeated hypoxic events during infancy and a possible impairment of neural function is well documented (Deykin et al 1984, Löscher et al 1990, Einspieler 1994, Einspieler et al 1994, Einspieler 1995, Kahn et al 1996). The largest study so far on this topic reported a high correlation between prolonged apnoeas and an impairment of the quality of spontaneous movements, including GMs, in 114 infants, aged between 3 and 26 weeks (Einspieler 1994).

Term infants with repeated and prolonged apnoeas during sleep may have poor repertoire GMs, even incidentally cramped GMs, but seldom tremulous GMs during their first two months. At 3 to 5 months, fidgety movements can be of abnormal exaggerated quality. Together with a poor attention to the environment, some infants may have a markedly reduced movement repertoire and even stereotypies.

Brain malformations
GMs are present but abnormal in infants with anencephaly (fronto-nasal encephalocele), parieto-occipital encephalocele, hydrocephaly, hydranencephaly, polymicrogyria, holoprosencephaly, hemimegaloencephaly, macrocephaly and microcephaly (Ferrari et al 1997). However, several other spontaneous movement patterns usually present in normal young infants are lacking (for the normal repertoire see Chapter 2). Isolated arm or leg movements were not observed in the infants with anencephaly, hydranencephaly, holoprosencephaly, macrocephaly and microcephaly. The infant with polymicrogyria and the infant with microcephaly did not have startles. The infant with a parieto-occipital encephalocele never rotated the head. No relationship was observed between the defective movement patterns and specific brain malformation (Ferrari et al 1997).

The temporal organisation of the GMs was clearly abnormal in the infant with anencephaly and the infant with macrocephaly (pachygyria and cerebellum hypoplasia). The GMs occurred in burst–pause patterns instead of being scattered over the one-hour recording. Similar findings were observed in six out of eight anencephalic foetuses (Visser et al 1985).

Unusual postures were described for the majority of infants with brain malformations (Ferrari et al 1997). None of these cases showed the variability of postures described for the healthy infant (Cioni et al 1989).

As expected, all infants with distinct brain malformations exhibit abnormal movements. The study by Ferrari et al (1997) failed to demonstrate any connection between the degree of tissue loss and the degree of GM abnormality expressed by the GM optimality score (Ferrari et al 1990; see Fig. 3.8). Anencephaly and hydranencephaly were the two cases with the most defective brain tissue, yet the GM optimality score was not worse than in microcephaly, holoprosencephaly and other brain malformations with less defective brain tissue (Ferrari et al 1997).

ANENCEPHALY, FRONTO-NASAL ENCEPHALOCELE
The GM assessment revealed a variety of distinct abnormal GMs during the same recording (Fig. 6.15). Myoclonic jerks were superimposed on GMs (Ferrari et al 1997).

PARIETO-OCCIPITAL ENCEPHALOCELE
The monotony of the movement sequence was rather marked during term age. Fidgety movements were absent, but the motor repertoire consisted of cramped, repetitive, even synchronised movements of all limbs (Fig. 6.16). There were no movements towards the midline (Ferrari et al 1997).

CHROMOSOMAL ABNORMALITY [DEL(4)(P15.1)] AND CONGENITAL ASYMMETRICAL HYDROCEPHALUS
The GMs of a patient, born at 42 weeks, were of poor repertoire and floppy. At the 43-week recording a monotonous repetition of exo-rotations of the arms and fragmented limb

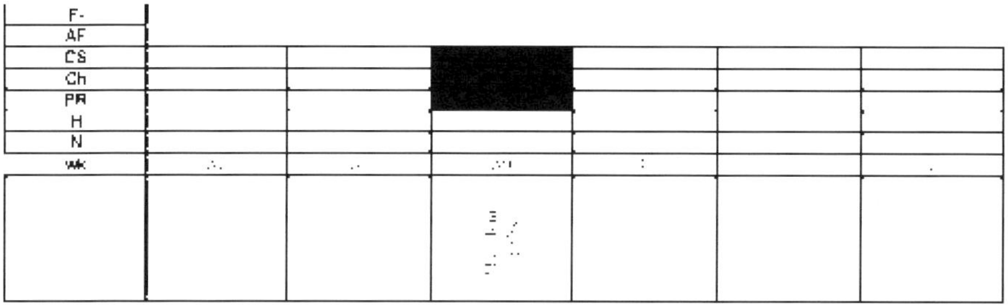

Fig. 6.15 GM assessment of case 21 born at 38 weeks postmenstrual age. Extension of brain tissue and cerebrospinal fluid through a defect in the skull base in the region of the cribriform plate and crista galli (computer tomography at 1 month); hypoplasia of the parietal bones of the skull, marked cerebrum hypoplasia, minimal shrinkage of the hemispheres, thinning of the cortex of the cerebellum, which was of normal size. Chaotic, cramped-synchronised and poor repertoire GMs at 39 weeks. Outcome: died at 4 months (Ferrari et al 1997). Abbreviations as in Fig. 6.1.

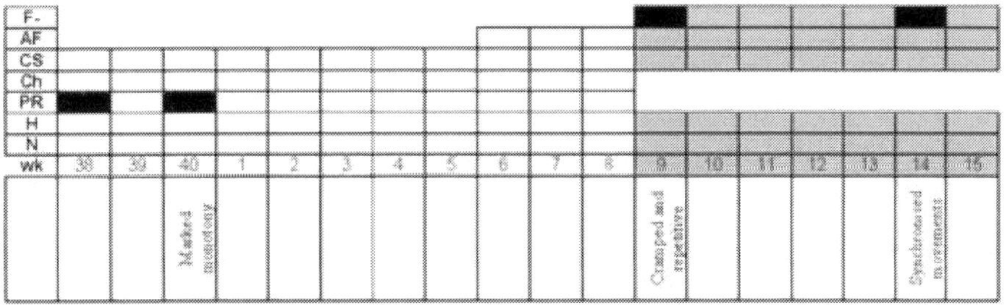

Fig. 6.16 Individual developmental trajectory of case 22 born at 36 weeks postmenstrual age. Vast occipital meningo-encephalocele, hyperintensity of its parenchymal part in T2-weighted images (MRI at 4 months). Poor repertoire GMs, absence of fidgety movements. Outcome: lost at the age of 11 months (Ferrari et al 1997). Abbreviations as in Fig. 6.1.

movements were observed. In addition, the infant had an unusual preference posture with a scoliosis of the neck and retroflexion of the head. The patient died at 2 months (Ferrari et al 1997).

HYDRANENCEPHALY

Fig. 6.17 demonstrates the longitudinal inconsistency of abnormal writhing movements in a patient with hydranencephaly.

POLYMICROGYRIA AND MULTIPLE MALFORMATIONS

In addition to polymicrogyria the patient (born at 41 weeks postmenstrual age) had a left eye coloboma and agenesis of the olfactory bulbs. GMs were recorded at 5 weeks postterm age and were scored as poor repertoire GMs due to the repetition of the same sequence. The patient died at 2 months of age (Ferrari et al 1997).

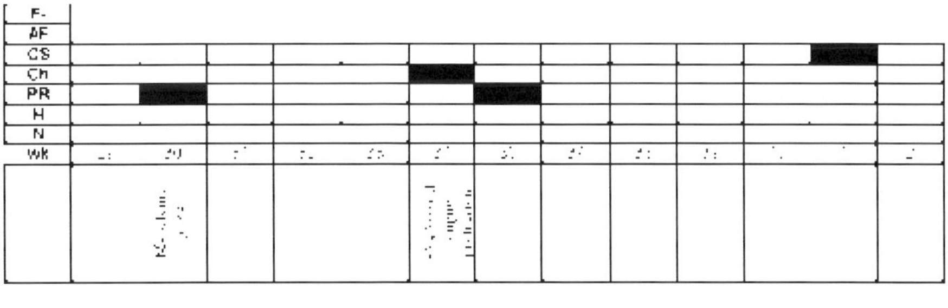

Fig. 6.17 Individual developmental trajectory of case 23 born at 25 weeks postmenstrual age. Hydranencephaly, cerebral hemispheres nearly completely replaced by cerebrospinal fluid; a minimal portion of the right fronto-temporal, right and left occipital lobes is conserved, thalami and cerebellum are present (MRI at 33 weeks postmenstrual age). Poor repertoire, chaotic and cramped-synchronised GMs. Outcome (3 years): macrocephaly, severe learning disability, spastic tetraplegia, blindness (Ferrari et al 1997). Abbreviations as in Fig. 6.1.

55

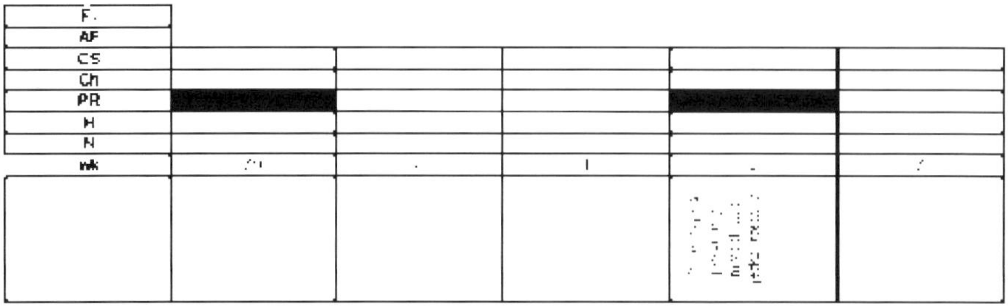

Fig. 6.18 GM assessment of case 24 born at 39 weeks postmenstrual age. Corpus callosum, falx cerebri and interhemispheric fissure agenesis, fused thalami, third ventricle not present, a crescent-shaped holoventricle surrounds fused thalami, pachygyria, marked thinning of the hemispheric white matter (MRI at 2 weeks); microcephaly, bilateral agenesis of the olfactory bulbs, frontal lobes fused by means of meninges, a shrimp of separation of the hemispheres is detectable, pachygyria, bilateral hypoplasia of the parietal and occipital lobe. Poor repertoire GMs. Outcome: died at 8 months (Ferrari et al 1997). Abbreviations as in Fig. 6.1.

HOLOPROSENCEPHALY

Despite a marked monotony of the movement sequence, elegant wrist rotations were observed in a term-age patient with holoprosencephaly. Three weeks later the poor repertoire was marked (Fig. 6.18). In addition, frequent asymmetric tonic neck postures, stereotyped pedalling, short-lasting limb movements, small in amplitude and similar to myoclonic jerks, and tremor occurred (Ferrari et al 1997).

HEMIMEGALOENCEPHALY

The writhing GMs of a patient born at term age were scored as poor repertoire. The patient had a marked magnification of the right hemisphere with thickening of the cortex. The right frontal lobe was normal (on magnetic resonance imaging at 2 weeks). After a right hemispherectomy at 12 months, the patient developed a left hemiplegia and learning disability (Ferrari et al 1997).

MACROCEPHALY

GM assessment of a patient with macrocephaly revealed a poor repertoire of writhing GMs (at 3 weeks postterm age) with additional tremulous movements. The onset of the movements was brisk and synchronised. From time to time brisk head rotations were observed. A week later the GMs were cramped-synchronised and still tremulous (Fig. 6.19). The opening of the mouth was synchronised with the limb movements (Ferrari et al 1997).

CONGENITAL MICROCEPHALY

The writhing GMs of a patient with congenital microcephaly (born at 38 weeks post-menstrual age) were scored as poor repertoire. In addition, repetitive rowing and pedalling movements, stereotyped adduction–abduction of the forearms, and abrupt and jerky head rotations were observed. Crying did not change the movement pattern. The patient developed severe learning disability (Ferrari et al 1997).

56

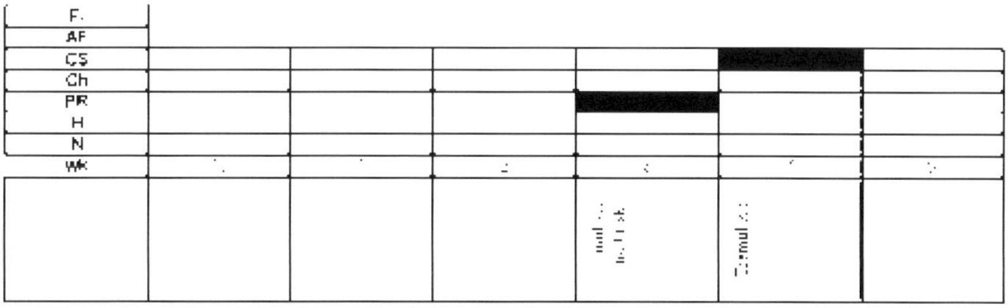

F.						
AF						
CS				▮		
Ch						
PR			▮			
H						
N						
wk	.	.	.	.	.	.
			mal b.·1>t.	·:mul<.:		

Fig. 6.19 GM assessment of case 25 born at 40 weeks postmenstrual age. Occipital horn of the lateral ventricles dilatated, corpus callosum hypoplasia (computer tomography at 4 weeks); macrocephaly and pachygyria, corpus callosum and cerebellum hypoplasia, dilatated lateral ventricles, delayed myelination. Poor repertoire and cramped-synchronised GMs. Outcome: died at 10 months (Ferrari et al 1997). Abbreviations as in Fig. 6.1.

No infant displayed GMs similar to those of another infant. With the exception of the anencephalic patient, the repetition of the same sequence within a GM or from GM to GM is the common feature of the brain malformed infant. Hence, the putative role of the forebrain structures in modulating the GM quality seems to be confirmed by the observation in these infants.

Spina bifida aperta

Recently, the quality of GMs was investigated in 20 term newborns with spina bifida aperta (Sival et al 2003). GMs were normal in eight infants and abnormal in nine (poor repertoire GMs in eight and cramped-synchronised GMs in one infant), while three infants were hypokinetic. There was a positive correlation between higher thoraco-lumbar myelomeningocoeles and abnormal GMs. In spina bifida aperta, the spinal defect (myelomeningocoele) often coexists with cerebral malformations such as Arnold–Chiari malformation, hydrocephalus, and corpus callosum hypoplasia. No relationship, however, between these brain malformations and the quality of GMs was found. The authors suggest that the abnormal qualitative characteristics of GMs in infants with higher thoraco-lumbar myelomeningocoeles relate to a more functionally impaired condition of the brain or brainstem.

Rett syndrome

Rett syndrome is due to an X-linked dominant disorder caused by mutations in a gene encoding methyl-CpG-binding protein 2 (Amir et al 1999). This protein binds to methylated DNA and may function as a transcriptional repressor by associating with the DNA chromatin-remodelling complexes. The resulting syndrome begins in seemingly normal 6- to 18-month-old infants and causes profound cognitive impairment. The cognitive impairment occurs without significant neurodegeneration but rather with a reduction in neuronal size (Bauman et al 1995), loss of dendritic development (Armstrong 1992, Armstrong et al 1995) and neuropile throughout grey matter areas in conjunction with a decrease in white matter (Akbarian 2002).

TABLE 6.1
Developmental course of fidgety movements in Rett syndrome (Einspieler et al 2004)

Quality of fidgety movements	End of 2nd month N = 12	3 to 4 months N = 10	5 to 6 months N = 11
Normal	0	0	0
Jerky, fast and disorganised	3	3	1
Jerky and slow	2	4	4
Absent as an abnormal sign	–	3	–
Not yet or no longer present	7	–	6

An apparently normal prenatal and perinatal period followed by an apparently normal psychomotor development during the first six months of life were considered as criteria for classical Rett syndrome (Hagberg et al 1983, Trevarthen and Moser 1988, Kerr 1995). However, several investigators consider it to be a developmental disorder manifesting at or very soon after birth (Witt-Engerström 1987, Naidu et al 1995, Percy 1995).

Recently, movements, posture and behaviour of 22 girls with Rett syndrome during their first half-year of life were carefully assessed from family videos. As well as a number of peculiar signs (e.g. abnormal finger movements, asymmetric eye opening and closing, bizarre smiling, bursts of abnormal facial expressions), all cases had abnormal GMs.

Writhing movements were of a poor repertoire. Some infants had predominant jerky and fast movements; others moved in slow motion and seemed to almost get stuck in their movement sequence. None of the 12 infants who were recorded during the fidgety movement period showed normal fidgety movements (Table 6.1). In addition, five infants already showed their abnormal fidgety movements at the end of their second month. Fidgety movements had disappeared unusually early – at 4 months – in six other infants.

The fact that none of the Rett cases had normal fidgety movements confirms the finding that normal fidgety movements are highly predictive for normal development (Prechtl et al 1997b). The absence of fidgety movements is clearly predictive for the spastic and dyskinetic forms of cerebral palsy (see Chapter 5). Interestingly enough, those infants with Rett syndrome without fidgety movements did not develop either hypertonicity or dystonic features. The abnormal quality of fidgety movements in infants with Rett syndrome is clearly different from the abnormal fidgety movements observed in infants with brain lesions, which are exaggerated with regard to their amplitude, speed and jerkiness (see Chapter 2). The fidgety movements of infants with Rett syndrome are jerky and are exhibited as either disorganised or in slow motion (Einspieler et al 2004).

Intra-uterine growth retardation
Intra-uterine growth retardation (IUGR) due to placental dysfunction is a risk factor for an impaired neurodevelopmental outcome (Allen 1984, Teberg et al 1988). This is the case particularly in growth-retarded foetuses whose conditions in utero are so compromised that they have to be delivered before term (Walther 1988, Sival et al 1992a).

Growth retardation is determined mostly on the basis of birth weight, and so IUGR is considered more or less equal to 'small for gestational age' (SGA). However, different criteria are used to define SGA. Some neonatologists define SGA as a birth weight below 5 (<P5) or 2.3 percentile (<P2.3) on a birth weight versus gestational age curve. Others regard all infants below the 10th percentile (<P10) as SGA. Especially if the broader criterion is applied, many of these infants would not qualify as intra-uterine growth-retarded at all; they just happen to fall into the lower range of the normal population distribution. In addition, some infants are born small because of an (undetected) chromosomal abnormality or dysmorphic syndrome. Finally, within the group of infants growth-restricted due to placental dysfunction, the onset and severity of the growth retardation add to the heterogeneity of the SGA group (Bos et al 2001).

Generally speaking, there is an increased risk for mild neurodevelopmental abnormalities with cognitive disabilities and behavioural problems, more so than for motor disturbances (Zubrick et al 2000). The risk for major neurological abnormalities in SGA infants is less clear. Several studies reported a slightly increased incidence of cerebral palsy, especially in term growth-retarded infants (Uvebrant and Hagberg 1992, Topp et al 1996), but also in preterm infants (Hadders-Algra et al 1988, Hagberg et al 1996).

In growth-retarded foetuses, a reduction in the quantity of GMs is a rather late sign of foetal deterioration (Bekedam et al 1985, 1987, Sival et al 1992a), since a reduction below the lower limit of normal only occurs in pre-terminal or terminal foetuses (Sival et al 1992a, Ribbert et al 1993). In SGA preterm infants, the rate of occurrence of various movement patterns did not differ from that found in low-risk preterm infants (Bos et al 1997c), with the exception of the duration of GMs during the first week after birth, which was significantly shorter in the SGA infants.

Several studies have investigated the quality of GMs in IUGR foetuses and infants. Movement quality was found to be impaired in IUGR foetuses (Bekedam et al 1985, Sival et al 1992b). Similar findings were reported in cross-sectional studies in preterm SGA infants (Geerdink and Hopkins 1993b) and fullterm SGA infants (van Kranen-Mastenbroek et al 1994).

The developmental course of the quality of GMs in preterm SGA infants has also been investigated. A clear relationship exists between specific developmental trajectories of GM quality and the neurological outcome at 2 years of age (Bos et al 1997b). However, the neurological outcome was not correlated to brain ultrasound findings, obstetrical variables indicative of foetal distress, the degree of growth retardation or the extent of brain sparing.It appears that most IUGR infants have an abnormal quality of GMs during their preterm period, but the longitudinal approach reveals that the quality of GMs normalises in the majority of the infants, albeit at or after term age (Bos et al 1997b). Fig. 6.20 demonstrates GM normalisation around term age followed by a normal neurological outcome.

A large proportion of foetuses and infants have slow motion GMs (Sival et al 1992b, Bos et al 1997b). In addition to the poor repertoire the GMs are predominantly slow with a small amplitude. They can precede a normalisation of GMs and hence a normal outcome (Fig. 6.21) or a deterioration of GMs and an impaired outcome (Fig. 6.22).

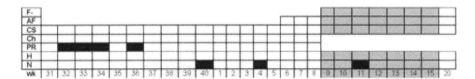

Fig. 6.20 Individual developmental trajectory of case 26 born at 31.4 weeks postmenstrual age, birth weight: 1010 grams; standard deviation score for birth weight: –1.89; percentage of brain weight: 16.7 (Cooke et al 1977); pregnancy-induced hypertension; pulsatility index of the umbilical artery: absent diastolic flow (Reuwer et al 1987); placenta: ischaemia 15 per cent infarction, weight < P3. Brain ultrasound: GMH-IVH grade 1 (Volpe 1989); periventricular leukomalacia grade 1 (de Vries LS et al 1992); duration of flares: three weeks. Poor repertoire GMs during the preterm period; normalisation around term age. Outcome (24 months): normal (Bos et al 1997b). Abbreviations as in Fig. 6.1.

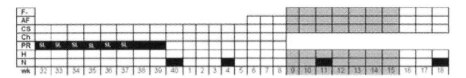

Fig. 6.21 Individual developmental trajectory of case 27 born at 32 weeks postmenstrual age, birth weight: 1115 grams; standard deviation score for birth weight: –1.65; percentage of brain weight: 16.8 (Cooke et al 1977); pulsatility index of the umbilical artery: absent diastolic flow (Reuwer et al 1987); late foetal heart rate deceleration; placenta: ischaemia 30 per cent infarction, weight < P3. Brain ultrasound: GMH-IVH grade 1 right (Volpe 1989); periventricular leukomalacia grade 1 (de Vries LS et al 1992); duration of flares: three weeks. Poor repertoire and slow motion (SL) GMs during the preterm period; normalisation at term age. Outcome (24 months): normal (Bos et al 1997b). Abbreviations as in Fig. 6.1.

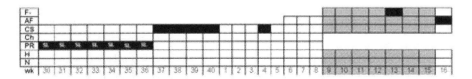

Fig 6.22 Individual developmental trajectory of case 28 born at 29.4 weeks postmenstrual age, birth weight: 840 grams; standard deviation score for birth weight: –1.92; percentage of brain weight: 16.2 (Cooke et al 1977); placenta: chorio-amnionitis. Brain ultrasound: occipital horns enlarged, prenatal onset. Poor repertoire and slow motion (SL) GMs followed by cramped-synchronised GMs, no fidgety movements at 13 weeks postterm and abnormal fidgety movements at 16 weeks. Outcome (24 months): neurologically abnormal, poor co-ordination (Bos et al 1997b). Abbreviations as in Fig. 6.1.

Chaotic GMs are frequently observed in growth-retarded infants (Figs 6.23 and 6.24), but have not been reported in growth-retarded foetuses (Bos et al 2001). In fullterm SGA infants, the qualitative assessment of movement patterns revealed an increased incidence of jerky and tremulous movements (van Kranen-Mastenbroek et al 1994). In preterm SGA infants, the presence of this abnormal movement pattern was related to late foetal heart-rate

60

decelerations and ischaemic alterations of the placenta (Bos et al 1997b). This indicates that acute foetal deterioration, superimposed on chronic placental insufficiency, might be responsible for the occurrence of this movement type. Chaotic GMs in SGA infants are not related to detectable brain lesions (Bos et al 2001).

It must be noted that cramped-synchronised GMs occur, if at all, postnatally rather late in growth-retarded infants (Fig. 6.22; Bos et al 2001). As demonstrated in Figs 6.21 to 6.24, the quality of fidgety movements, in particular, is predictive for the final outcome.

Interestingly, a large proportion of growth-retarded infants who have abnormal GMs have normal findings on brain ultrasound scans. This suggests that the chronically reduced foetal supply of oxygen and nutrients may lead to a longer-lasting but often transient brain dysfunction, which is not necessarily caused by haemorrhagic or hypoxic-ischaemic lesions detectable on ultrasound scans (Bos et al 1997b).

A final point deserves mentioning. The qualitative assessment of GMs has proved its worth mainly in relation to the prediction of motor disorders. Future studies will need to elucidate whether the quality of GMs is also predictive for the cognitive disabilities and behavioural problems which are found more often in IUGR infants (Bos et al 2001).

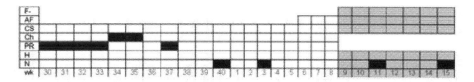

Fig. 6.23 Individual developmental trajectory of case 29 born at 28.7 weeks postmenstrual age, birth weight: 640 grams; standard deviation score for birth weight: –1.97; percentage of brain weight: 22.7 (Cooke et al 1977); pulsatility index of the umbilical artery: increased (Reuwer et al 1987); late foetal heart rate deceleration; placenta: severe ischaemia, retroplacental haematoma, no infarction, weight P3–P10. Brain ultrasound: GMH-IVH grade 2 right (Volpe 1989); periventricular leukomalacia grade 1 (de Vries LS et al 1992); duration of flares: four weeks. Poor repertoire GMs followed by chaotic GMs, normalisation at term age. Outcome (24 months): normal (Bos et al 1997b). Abbreviations as in Fig. 6.1.

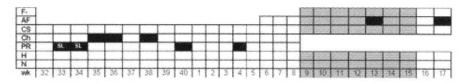

Fig. 6.24 Individual developmental trajectory of case 30 born at 32.1 weeks postmenstrual age, birth weight: 810 grams; standard deviation score for birth weight: –2.65; percentage of brain weight: 21.7 (Cooke et al 1977); pregnancy-induced hypertension; pulsatility index of the umbilical artery: increased (Reuwer et al 1987); late foetal heart rate deceleration; placenta: not known. Brain ultrasound: normal. Poor repertoire and slow motion GMs followed by chaotic GMs, abnormal fidgety movements. Outcome (24 months): abnormal neurological findings, poor coordination, habitual toe walking (Bos et al 1997b). Abbreviations as in Fig. 6.1.

Maternal diabetes mellitus

Foetuses of women with type-I diabetes are at increased risk for malformation, macrosomia, and impaired development of the central nervous system (Jovanovic et al 1981, Laurini et al 1984, Mulder 1992, Rizzo et al 1994, Persson and Hanson 1996, Nelson et al 2000, Penney et al 2003).

In a longitudinal study on twelve cases, foetal GMs were analysed at two-weekly intervals from 16 weeks postmenstrual age onwards and after birth during the first, second and third to fourth month (Kainer et al 1997). Foetal hyperinsulinism might cause foetal hypoxia (MacFarlane and Tsakalakos 1985, Petry et al 1994), and correlates with abnormal GMs, i.e. poor repertoire GMs or abrupt, jerky and fragmented GMs (Kainer et al 1997). As foetal hyperinsulinism may develop despite satisfactory maternal metabolic control, the latter is no guarantee against developmental disorders. Abnormal foetal GMs have always been associated with abnormal postnatal GMs (poor repertoire writhing movements and abnormal fidgety movements) and a reduced Bayley (1969) score at 10 months. On the other hand, normal foetal GMs may be followed by abnormal postnatal GMs if difficulties during delivery lead to neurological dysfunctions (Kainer et al 1997).

Early blindness

For a better understanding of the contribution vision makes to the development of other sensory systems and to movement and posture, we studied the effects of early blindness by examining lengthy and repeated video recordings of 14 totally blind infants. The infants were born either at term or preterm and showed no evidence of brain damage (Prechtl et al 2001).

As in sighted infants, the early blind infant showed complex, fluent and frequently occurring GMs prior to the third month of age. No differences were observed for isolated arm and leg movements, stretches, yawns, trunk and head rotations, nor for short phasic movements such as startles and twitches (Prechtl et al 2001).

A very striking feature concerned a peculiar type of fidgety movement. In all blind infants, observed during the relevant age range, fidgety movements were grossly disturbed in a specific way. They were exaggerated in amplitude and jerky in character and their presence lasted longer than in sighted infants. In fact, they were observed until 8 to 10 months postterm age (Prechtl et al 2001). Moreover, these movements were distinctly different from the abnormal fidgety movements seen in some brain-damaged infants (see Chapter 2).

In order to investigate if actual visual control is necessary for normal fidgety movements, six 3-month-old sighted, awake infants were filmed in the dark with a special light-sensitive camera. Their fidgety movements did not change in character and continued to look normal. Experiments to blindfold these infants failed because they immediately protested by crying, which itself inhibits fidgety movements. Prechtl (1997a) conjectured that the period of normal fidgety movements is necessary to re-calibrate the proprioceptive system (see also Chapters 4 and 5). The observation of the early blind infants supports this hypothesis. We speculate that exaggerated fidgety movements may be indicative of an attempt to compensate for the lack of integration of proprioception and vision (Prechtl et al 2001).

7

QUANTITATIVE ASSESSMENT IS AN INSENSITIVE INDICATOR OF IMPAIRED INTEGRITY OF THE NERVOUS SYSTEM

There is a large range of intra-individual and inter-individual variability in the rate of movement patterns throughout pregnancy (de Vries JIP et al 1985, 1987, Roodenburg et al 1991). The same holds true for healthy preterm and fullterm infants (Prechtl et al 1979, Prechtl and Nolte 1984, Cioni et al 1989, Cioni and Prechtl 1990).

Perhaps biased by the keen interest of obstetricians in the quantity of foetal movements as an indicator of foetal well-being, it was originally expected that a decrease (or even an increase) in the quantity of postnatal motility might act as a reliable indicator of brain dysfunction. This expectation turned out to be wrong. The large scatter in the quantitative data of spontaneous motility in uncompromised foetuses and in healthy infants makes quantitative assessment an insensitive indicator of compromising conditions of the nervous system.

Prechtl and Nolte (1984) compared quantitative data of 14 low-risk preterm infants with data of 13 infants of a high-risk group and failed to find differences. This was corroborated by Ferrari et al (1990) who compared the rate of movement patterns such as startles, GMs (Fig. 7.1), isolated arm and leg movements, twitches, cloni and tremulous movements in 12 matched pairs of preterm infants with and without brain lesion, respectively. An interesting finding was that even the comparison of the occurrence of tremulous movements reached only borderline significance ($p = 0.06$, Wilcoxon text for matched pairs; Ferrari et al 1990).

Other authors confirmed the lack of difference in the quantity (frequency and duration) of various movement patterns between a high-risk group with brain lesion and subsequent disability, and a low-risk group developing normally (Hines et al 1980, Erkinjuntti 1988).

In growth-retarded preterm infants, the rate of occurrence of various movement patterns did not differ from that found in low-risk preterm infants (Bos et al 1997c), with the exception of the duration of GMs during the first week after birth, which was significantly shorter in the growth-retarded infants (see Chapter 6). Hardly any correlations were found between the quantity of movement patterns after birth and obstetrical variables indicative of a compromised foetal condition. Only a reduction in foetal heart rate variation was found to correlate slightly with an increased incidence of startles and twitches in the first week after birth (Bos et al 1997c).

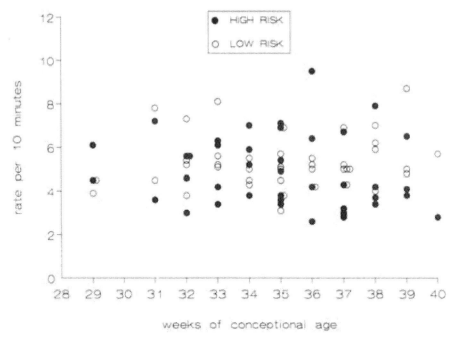

Fig. 7.1 Longitudinal comparison of the incidence of GMs (rate per 10 minutes) in 12 matched pairs of preterm infants with and without brain lesion, respectively (reproduced with permission from Ferrari et al 1990).

Even in severely brain-malformed foetuses (Visser et al 1985) and infants (Ferrari et al 1997), qualitative changes in spontaneous movements prevailed over quantitative changes. As for the quantitative abnormalities of spontaneous movements, in nine infants with various brain malformations, they consisted of the lack of one or more movement patterns (see Chapter 6). However, the defective movement pattern, or combination of patterns, was not related to specific brain abnormality or the severity of tissue loss (Ferrari et al 1997).

It is obvious that quantitative changes in motility are unsuitable markers of neurological dysfunction in foetuses and young infants. This is in striking contrast to the qualitative aspects of motility which change dramatically in the case of brain damage.

8
BRAIN ULTRASOUND AND GENERAL MOVEMENT ASSESSMENT

Brain ultrasound is the most frequently used imaging technique to detect structural changes in the newborn's brain and has been considered the best predictor of neurological outcome (Levene 1990). Studies on the relationship between ultrasound findings, developmental trajectories and neurological outcome revealed the GM assessment to be superior to ultrasound findings (Ferrari et al 1990, Cioni et al 1997a, 1997c, Prechtl 1997b, Bos 1998, Bos et al 1998a, Ferrari et al 2002). Case histories provided in Chapter 6 (Figs 6.3, 6.5, 6.6, 6.8, 6.10, 6.12, 6.13, 6.20, 6.21, 6.23, 6.24) illustrate the superior predictive power of longitudinal GM assessment as indicated by individual developmental trajectories.

The largest longitudinal study so far on GM assessment was carried out on 130 infants. Their ultrasound findings, ranging from normal to severely abnormal, were classified into two groups: 70 low-risk and 60 high-risk cases. Examples of abnormal ultrasound findings judged to be mild enough to allow classification into the low-risk group were short-lasting increased echogenicity or grade 1 intraventricular haemorrhage. High-risk infants were found to have definite abnormalities of their brains on ultrasound examination (periventricular leukomalacia grade 2 to 4 according to de Vries LS et al 1992, and grade 2 to 3 plus intra- and periventricular haemorrhage according to Volpe 1989). The sensitivity of the GM assessment during the first weeks of life (94 per cent) and of the assessment of fidgety movements (95 per cent) was higher than that of brain ultrasound imaging, which was 80 per cent. Specificity for GM assessment during the fidgety movement period was 96 per cent whereas for brain ultrasound it was 83 per cent (Prechtl et al 1997b).

Similar results were reported for 66 preterm and 58 fullterm infants (Cioni et al 1997a, 1997c). A recent study on 34 infants with cystic and 34 infants with non-cystic abnormalities of the white matter confirmed the high predictive power of GM assessment (Ferrari et al 2002). The receiver operating characteristic (ROC) curve analysis was used (Metz 1978) to compare the power of brain ultrasound (5 to 7.5 MHz heads) and GM assessment to predict cerebral palsy (Fig. 8.1). This method provides a powerful means of assessing a test's ability to discriminate between two groups of patients, with the advantage that analysis does not depend on the threshold value selected (Metz 1978).

The areas under the ROC curve analysis for GM assessment and ultrasound scans were quite large (97.4 and 88.3, respectively), which shows that they are both accurate tests. A statistically significant difference was found, however, between the two methods ($p < 0.001$), indicating that the GM assessment is a better index to predict neurological outcome in a group of infants who were selected on the basis of abnormal ultrasound findings (Ferrari et al 2002).

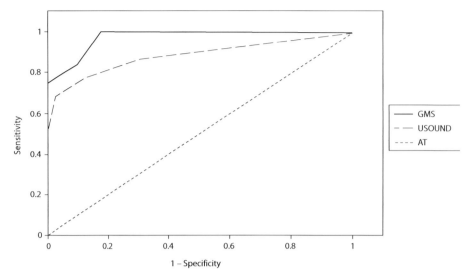

Fig. 8.1 The area under the receiver operating characteristic (ROC) curve for quality of GMs and ultrasound (USOUND) scans in high-risk preterm infants. The ROC curve is generated by plotting the proportion of true positive results against the proportion of false positive results for each value of a test. The curve for an arbitrary test (AT) that is expected to have no discriminatory value appears as a diagonal line, whereas a useful test has an ROC curve that rises rapidly and reaches a plateau (reproduced with permission from Ferrari et al 2002).

In infants with severe brain lesion, the longitudinal assessment of GMs (individual developmental trajectory) helps to distinguish those infants who have a fair prognosis from those who have not. For infants with minor ultrasound abnormalities the GM assessment is particularly helpful and helps to identify those infants who are at risk for developmental problems and those who are not (Prechtl 1997a, Bos 1998). We have to bear in mind that during the last few years brain ultrasound equipment and assessment have improved considerably.

Of course, GM assessment can never replace neuroimaging techniques but it is a worthwhile method to be used in combination with neuroimaging. This has also been illustrated by two studies on GM assessment and neonatal magnetic resonance imaging (Cioni et al 2000, Guzzetta et al 2003). Another recent study on term infants with hypoxic ischaemic encephalopathy demonstrated that the combined use of GM assessment and proton magnetic resonance spectroscopy (1H MRS) increases the prognostic value (Rapisardi et al 2002).

9
NEUROLOGICAL EXAMINATION AND GENERAL MOVEMENT ASSESSMENT

The introduction of sophisticated neuroimaging techniques has supplemented but not replaced the neurological examination of the newborn. The information provided by this examination is still very important for a rapid diagnosis of a neurological disorder in a newborn, for deciding on the need for and type of imaging, electrophysiological or other examinations to be carried out, for formulating a prognosis and for monitoring, by repeated checks, the development of the disorder (Cioni et al 1997c).

Since the first description of concepts and criteria for the neurological examination of newborns by André Thomas and Saint-Anne Dargassies (1952), several protocols have been published. However, only two comprehensive methods of neonatal neurological examination have been standardised and validated, those of Prechtl (1977, Prechtl and Beintema 1964) for term infants and of Dubowitz and Dubowitz (1981, Dubowitz et al 1999) for both term and preterm infants.

A systematic comparison of the qualitative assessment of GMs and the traditional neurological examination in selected groups of preterm and term infants revealed the superior predictive power of the assessment of GMs for all age groups, but particularly at the younger ages (Cioni et al 1997a, 1997c, Ferrari et al 2002).

The preterm infant
Preterm infants are generally submitted to a neurological examination in the neonatal period, with the aim of assessing the functional consequences of brain lesion, which may have been found by neuroimaging, and to predict long-term neurological outcome. It is always preferable to use a comprehensive, structured and standardised neurological examination than a random selection of items. Standardised and validated protocols permit testing the different subsystems of the neonatal nervous system. For the preterm period the protocol by Dubowitz and Dubowitz (1981; new edition: Dubowitz et al 1999) is available. It is difficult to apply some of the Dubowitz items to fragile preterms (Cioni et al 1997a) and the predictive values are rather low (Dubowitz et al 1984, Molteno et al 1995).

In a comparative study on 66 preterm infants with various brain ultrasound findings (from normal to grade 3 intraventricular haemorrhage and periventricular leukomalacia) the percentage of agreement (normal versus abnormal) between GM assessment and neurological examination during the preterm period was quite low, namely 73 per cent. As these

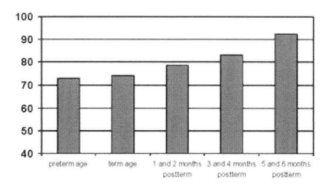

Fig. 9.1 Percentage of agreement between GM assessment and neurological examination at preterm age according to Dubowitz and Dubowitz (1981), at term age according to Prechtl (1977), at the postterm period according to Amiel-Tison and Grenier (1983) and Touwen (1976), reported by Cioni et al (1997a).

infants were repeatedly examined, the percentage of agreement constantly increased, reaching 92.6 per cent at the 4- to 5-month-examination (Fig. 9.1). Overall agreement was 80 per cent (Cioni et al 1997a).

The sensitivity of the GM assessment is very high at all ages (Fig. 9.2), but the specificity is low during the preterm, term and early postterm period (Fig. 9.3). This is due to a consistent number of infants with abnormal GMs who normalise during the fidgety movement period and have a normal outcome (see also Chapter 5). Thus, specificity only becomes high at 3 to 4 months.

The sensitivity of the neurological examination is quite low at preterm and term age, because of infants with apparently normal findings during their neurological examination who develop cerebral palsy (Fig. 9.2). In the first postnatal weeks, physical conditions

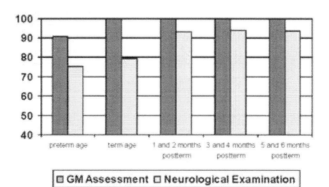

Fig. 9.2 Sensitivity (in %) of GM assessment and neurological examination at preterm age according to Dubowitz and Dubowitz (1981), at term age according to Prechtl (1977), at the postterm period according to Amiel-Tison and Grenier (1983) and Touwen (1976), with respect to an abnormal neurological outcome at 2 years (Cioni et al 1997a).

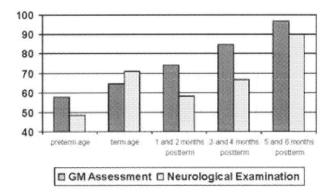

Fig. 9.3 Specificity (in %) of GM assessment and neurological examination at preterm age according to Dubowitz and Dubowitz (1981), at term age according to Prechtl (1977), at the postterm period according to Amiel-Tison and Grenier (1983) and Touwen (1976), with respect to a normal neurological outcome at 2 years (Cioni et al 1997a).

(e.g. anaemia, jaundice, apnoeas, cardiac instability) might account for poor responses at the neurological examination and its failure in terms of long-term prediction of disabilities. At term, some infants who later develop spastic diplegia show a normal neurological examination. As mentioned by Dubowitz (1988), this might be due to transient normalisation of the muscle tonus while changing from preterm hypotonia to postterm hypertonia. The specificity for the neurological examination is low until 4 months (Fig. 9.3).

The very high sensitivity for the GM assessment right from preterm age onwards is mainly due to cramped-synchronised GMs and their high predictive value for cerebral palsy (Ferrari et al 1990, 2002; see also Chapter 5). A recent comparison between GM assessment and neurological examination of 84 preterm infants replicated and confirmed the results provided in Figs 9.2 and 9.3 (Ferrari et al 2002).

In addition, a four-centre study on preterm infants with unilateral intraparenchymal echodensity replicated also the superior predictive power of longitudinal GM assessment. Particularly at preterm and term age, neurological examination had a higher number of false-negatives and false-positives for the neurological outcome than the GM assessment. Moreover, the three cases with unilateral intraparenchymal echodensity who did not develop hemiplegia had normal fidgety movements, although one of them had abnormal findings at the neurological examination, i.e. hypertonia and asymmetry (Cioni et al 2000).

The authors of the above-mentioned studies recommended caution in the comparison of GM assessment and neurological examination. The units involved in the studies used different protocols for the neurological examination, namely those adopted in their daily practice. The GM observation, however, had the advantage of being carried out subsequently from video recordings and was certainly more consistent.

The fullterm infant

A first comparison between GM assessment and neurological examination in fullterm infants with hypoxic-ischaemic encephalopathy indicated a slightly higher prognostic value of GM assessment in the first two weeks postterm and of neurological examination at about 5 to 6 months (Prechtl et al 1993).

The first systematic comparison was carried out on 58 infants (Cioni et al 1997c) representing uneventful obstetrical and neonatal histories as well as hypoxic-ischaemic encephalopathy of various degrees according to a three-point grading system (Levene et al 1982). The neurological examination at the various ages (Touwen 1976, Prechtl 1977, Amiel-Tison and Grenier 1983) resulted in more abnormal findings than did the GM assessment. The overall percentage of agreement was 81 per cent and thus similar to that in preterm infants (Cioni et al 1997a; see Fig. 9.1).

GM assessment and neurological examination had good sensitivity values (Table 9.1), slightly better for the former at all age periods. Specificity was low for both techniques at term age, because some subjects with poor repertoire GMs or mild neurological abnormalities at that age were normal at 2 years. At 2 months postterm the specificity for the GM assessment was good and already superior to the neurological examination (Table 9.1). According to these data, normalisation of transient disorders might be assessed earlier by GM observation (Fig. 9.4).

A lower agreement between GM assessment and neurological examination was reported by Hadders-Algra et al (1997). However, the number of cases included in that study was quite small (16 cases), no distinction between term and preterm infants was made for the comparison, and a more elaborate classification of GM abnormalities was applied, distinguishing more different categories (see Chapter 10).

According to these findings, the prognostic value of the GM assessment in fullterm infants also is superior to the neurological examination. However, there are limitations to the application of GM assessment. In infants with severe hypoxic-ischaemic encephalopathy, in their first hours after birth neuroimaging, electrophysiological techniques,

TABLE 9.1
Predictive values of GM assessment and neurological examination (Touwen 1976,
Prechtl 1977, Amiel-Tison and Grenier 1983) with respect to the neurological outcome
at 2 years in 58 term-born infants (Cioni et al 1997c)

		Sensitivity		Specificity	
		GM assessment	Neurological examination	GM assessment	Neurological examination
Writhing movements	Term age	94%	88%	59%	59%
	1 and 2 months	94%	88%	86%	68%
Fidgety movements	3 and 4 months	94%	89%	83%	73%

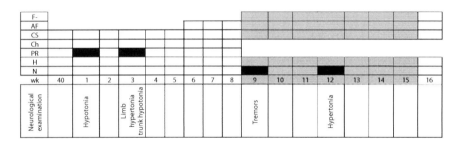

Fig 9.4 Individual developmental trajectory of case 31 born at 39 weeks postmenstrual age. GM assessment and neurological examination (Touwen 1976, Prechtl 1977, Amiel-Tison and Grenier 1983). Brain ultrasound: periventricular leukomalacia grade 2, bright thalami. GM assessment: poor repertoire followed by normal fidgety movements. Neurological examination: abnormal findings until 12 weeks postterm. Outcome (24 months): normal (Cioni et al 1997c).

F-, absence of fidgety movements; AF, abnormal fidgety movements; CS, cramped-synchronised GMs; Ch, chaotic GMs; PR, poor repertoire GMs; H, hypokinesis; N, normal GMs; wk, weeks. The age period where fidgety movements are obligatory is marked in grey.

and some subtests of traditional clinical assessment have a prominent role in detecting the severity of brain impairment and indicating the prognosis (Eken et al 1995, Mercuri and Dubowitz 1996). Moreover, traditional neurological assessment provides a more comprehensive picture of the various neural subsystems, some of which (e.g. the oculo-motor system or peripheral nerves) cannot be tested by GM observation.

GM assessment clearly should complement but not replace the neurological examination. Both have different properties and diagnostic tasks (Prechtl 1997a).

10
WHAT OTHER METHODS OF GENERAL MOVEMENT ASSESSMENT EXIST?

There are a number of reports which are based on different criteria of qualitative assessment of early spontaneous motility.

Touwen (1990) did not focus on a particular movement pattern but classified the quality 'of movements' according to three paired categories: patterned versus unpatterned and isolated; smooth versus jerky; and variable versus stereotyped or monotonous.

With his classification scheme Touwen observed 47 preterm infants between 33 and 36 weeks postmenstrual age. Motility is classified as 'patterned' when the movement patterns are consistently composite and recognisable. The movements involve either the whole body or only single parts, such as an arm or a leg. They must consist of more than one component; a single flexion of the arm is not considered to be a pattern but a flexion-extension movement is. 'Isolated movements' are limited to single joints and consist of, for example, just an extension of the arm not followed by a flexion. If no consistent pattern can be recognised, motility is termed 'chaotic' or 'erratic'; this, however, occurs rarely (Touwen 1990).

Movements are termed 'smooth' when they are uninterrupted, continuous and fluent 'with gradual accelerations and decelerations' similar to how Prechtl and co-workers described normal GMs (Prechtl 1990). Movements termed 'jerky' are abrupt, oscillating or tremulous, with an interrupted, broken course and sudden accelerations and decelerations (Touwen 1990).

'Variable' movements denote changes in speed, amplitude and direction, as well as the presence of various patterns and postures. It implies a repertoire of movements, but also variations in the repertoire. 'Monotonous' motility is characterised by invariability in type, direction, speed and often amplitude of movements. There is a lack of variation in patterns and infants may persist in one – often rather poor – pattern for long periods. Persistent asymmetries or preferences in motility or posture are also considered to be stereotyped (Touwen 1990).

These three paired categories are summarised in a variable/stereotyped ratio, which could vary from 3/0 to 0/3. A high ratio correlates with a normal outcome whereas a low ratio is not predictive for the outcome (Touwen 1990). Data on interscorer agreement are not available.

Van Kranen-Mastenbroek and co-workers used general movements for their qualitative assessment but employed a different categorisation of normal and abnormal quality. The main difference lies in the attention to too many details instead of focusing primarily on a global Gestalt judgement. The latter is only used as the last item of the procedure. The other items are: onset of movement, variability in speed, overall speed, speed of arms compared to legs, force against gravity, variability in amplitude, overall amplitude, amplitude of arms compared to legs, fluency, variability in movement pattern, variability in arm patterns, variability in leg patterns, fine distal movements, and end of movement (van Kranen-Mastenbroek et al 1992, 1994). The agreement rates of four observers scoring 50 neonates ranged from kappa = 0.36 to 0.84, and were best for the global judgement (see also Chapter 5) and below 0.40 for 'amplitude', 'variability in movements' and 'variability in leg movements' (van Kranen-Mastenbroek et al 1992).

GM quality types I to V are distinguished. Type I GMs are similar to the normal GMs described by Prechtl (1990). Type II GMs are fast movements with an abrupt and jerky appearance. They are variable in speed and amplitude. Type III GMs are abrupt and jerky, have lost their variability and complexity and give a stereotyped impression. The speed is high and the amplitude is large. Type IV GMs are fluent with slow speed, but stereotyped. Type V GMs are tremulous, sometimes flapping, with a stereotyped character (van Kranen-Mastenbroek et al 1994).

Predictive values are based on 30 neonates and on an outcome measurement at 9 months indicating relationships between the GM assessment and the 9-month investigation (van Kranen-Mastenbroek et al 1994).

Hadders-Algra and co-workers introduced a new terminology and a considerably enlarged categorisation of the existing types of GM abnormalities, based on EMG recordings of six term-born and ten preterm-born infants. As well as normal GMs, which are defined according to Prechtl's definition (Prechtl 1990, Prechtl et al 1997a), Hadders-Algra et al (1997) distinguish between 'mildly abnormal GMs' and 'definitely abnormal GMs'.

Mildly abnormal GMs are split into 'fragmented' and 'tense' GMs. 'Fragmented GMs' are moderately complex and moderately variable with a jerky and broken appearance. They may give the impression of a reduced capacity to modulate movement speed and force. From 3 months onwards a fragmented form of fidgety movements can be observed. Fragmented fidgety movements lack the elegance of normal fidgety movements and are usually accompanied by a large amount of very rapid arm movements, so-called 'swats' (Hadders-Algra and Prechtl 1992), and kicking leg movements. 'Tense GMs' are also moderately complex and moderately variable GMs with a rather stiff appearance. The onset can be abrupt, but the ensuing movements are slow. The tense character is more strikingly present in the lower half than in the upper half of the body. A common observation is stiff legs sticking up in extension (Hadders-Algra et al 1997).

Definitely abnormal GMs are split into four categories. 'Torpid GMs' consist of slow-motion movements, which in general have a small amplitude. The movements give the impression that the drive to move is depressed. During torpid GMs rotations superimposed on flexion and extension movements can occasionally be observed. These movements are only present until 2 months postterm age. 'Monotonous-abrupt GMs' are predominated by abrupt and fast movements. In general, the movements of the limbs have a large amplitude. There is a characteristic repetition of similar abrupt and fast movements. They often elicit crying. 'Monotonous-cramped GMs' are monotonously stiff, rigid and very tense. They have an abrupt and synchronous onset of movement activity in all limbs and are obviously synonymous with the cramped-synchronised GMs of Prechtl's method. 'Monotonous GMs' are characterised by a complete lack of complexity and total absence of variation, but do not have an abrupt or cramped character (Hadders-Algra et al 1997).

By and large, the category of poor repertoire GMs of Prechtl's method is divided into four categories, namely fragmented, tense, torpid and monotonous GMs. With the exception of 'torpid GMs' all abnormal patterns can be observed from preterm age onwards including the fidgety movement period. Thus, Hadders-Algra and co-workers do not use any more the categorisation into abnormal fidgety movements or the highly predictive absence of fidgety movements. In addition, the terminology is interpretative (e.g. 'mildly abnormal', 'definitely abnormal') instead of descriptive.

Interscorer agreement ranged from kappa values of 0.53 up to 1.00. Validity data are provided for 16 children, two of whom were classified as normal at around 19 months.

Kakebeeke and co-workers used a ten-point scale based on the assessment of fluency, spatio-temporal variability and sequencing of GMs. Fluency and variability are separately assessed in arms and legs. The scoring system was applied in 39 preterm infants and 20 fullterm infants during their preterm and term period. Interscorer agreement was between 56 per cent, for sequencing, and 76 per cent, for leg variability (Kakebeeke et al 1997, 1998). No data on the predictive values are given.

The scoring of the quality of spontaneous movements is also included in the neurological assessment of the preterm and fullterm newborn infant by Dubowitz et al (1999). Fluent and alternating movements of arms and legs with a good variability are classed as optimal. Stretches alternating with fluent and smooth movements are classed as borderline, whereas only stretches, monotonous movements and cramped-synchronised movements are classed as suboptimal.

EPILOGUE

This book is an introduction to Prechtl's method on GM assessment. Training is needed for a proper application of this objective, reliable and valid method. In order to provide standardised training courses the General Movement Trust was founded in 1997. Heinz Prechtl (president of the Trust), Arend Bos, Christa Einspieler, Giovanni Cioni, Fabrizio Ferrari, Paola Paolicelli and Federica Roversi are licensed tutors for GM Trust training courses. These courses last four to five days and are aimed at physicians, physiotherapists and other professionals working in the field of infant neurology. They are regularly provided in English, German and Italian at a basic and advanced level. More than one thousand doctors and therapists have been trained around the world. The GM assessment is now widely employed in clinical routine. The high efficacy of these training courses is described in Chapter 6.

In addition to the DVD attached to this book, there is a demonstration video available (Prechtl 1997a). The video is published in English (contact: Dr Christa Einspieler, Fax: +43 316 380 9630; e-mail: christa.einspieler@meduni-graz.at), Italian (contact: Editrice Speciale Riabilitazione s.r.l., Fax: +39 02 54 116 227; e-mail: edspriab@tin.it), and Japanese (contact: Igakueizou Company, Fax: +81 3 3303 1434; http://www.igakueizou.co.jp; for a Japanese review see Yuge et al 2001 and Tsubokura 2002).

REFERENCES

Accardo PJ. (1997) Common sense. *J Pediatr* 130: 704–711.

Akbarian S. (2002) Rett's Syndrome, Part II. *Am J Psychiatr* 159: 1294. (Short communication.)

Albers S, Jorch G. (1994) Prognostic significance of spontaneous motility in very immature preterm infants under intensive care treatment. *Biol Neonat* 66: 182–187.

Alford S, Williams TL. (1989) Endogenous activation of glycine and NMDA receptors in lamprey spinal cord during fictive locomotion. *J Neurosci* 9: 2792–2800.

Allen MC. (1984) Developmental outcome and follow-up of the small for gestational age infant. *Sem Perinat* 8: 123–156.

Amiel-Tison C, Grenier A. (1983) *Neurologic Evaluation of the Newborn and the Infant*. New York: Masson.

Amir RE, van den Veyver IB, Wan M, Tran CQ, Francke U, Zoghbi HY. (1999) Rett syndrome is caused by mutations in X-linked MECP2, encoding methyl-CpG-binding protein 2. *Nature Gen* 23: 185–188.

Antri M, Orsal D, Barthe JY. (2002) Locomotor recovery in the chronic spinal rat: effects of long-term treatment with a 5-HT2 agonist. *Eur J Neurosci* 16: 467–476.

Armstrong D. (1992) The neuropathology of the Rett syndrome. *Brain Dev* 14: 89–98.

Armstrong D, Dunn JK, Antalffy B, Trivedi R. (1995) Selective dendritic alterations in the cortex of Rett syndrome. *J Neuropathol Exp Neurol* 54: 195–201.

Atkinson J. (1984a) How does infant vision change in the first three months of life? In: Prechtl HFR, editor. *Continuity of Neural Functions from Prenatal to Postnatal Life*. Clin Dev Med 94. Oxford: Blackwell, pp 159–178.

Atkinson J. (1984b) Human visual development over the first 6 months of life. A review and a hypothesis. *Hum Neurobiol* 3: 61–74.

Baarsma R, Laurini RN, Baerts W, Okken A. (1987) Reliability of sonography in non-haemorrhagic periventricular leukomalacia. *Pediatr Radiol* 17: 189–191.

Baldi I. (2002) The preterm infant with prolonged periventricular hyperechogenicity: prognostic role of neurological assessment and the effects of neonatal care (in Italian). Medical doctoral thesis, University of Pisa.

Bauman ML, Kemper TL, Arin DM. (1995) Microscopic observations of the brain in Rett syndrome. *Neuropediatrics* 26: 105–108.

Bax M. (2002) Clinical assessment still matters. *Dev Med Child Neurol* 44: 147. (Editorial.)

Bayley N. (1969) *Bayley Scales of Infant Development*. Berkeley: The Psychological Corporation.

Bekedam DJ, Visser GHA, de Vries JIP, Prechtl HFR. (1985) Motor behaviour in the growth retarded fetus. *Early Hum Dev* 12: 173–182.

Bekedam DJ, Visser GHA, Mulder EJH, Poelmann-Weesjes G. (1987) Heart rate variation and movement incidence in growth-retarded fetuses: the significance of antenatal late heart rate decelerations. *Am J Obstet Gynecol* 157: 126–133.

Birnholz JC. (1981) The development of human fetal eye movement patterns. *Science* 213: 679–681.

Bland M. (1996) *An Introduction to Medical Statistics*. Oxford: Medical Publications.

Bobath B. (1971) *Abnormal Postural Reflex Activity Caused by Brain Lesions*. London: Heinemann.

Bos AF. (1993) Differential effects of brain lesions and systemic disease on the quality of general movements: a preliminary report. *Early Hum Dev* 34: 39–45.

Bos AF. (1998) Analysis of movement quality in preterm infants. *Eur J Obstet Gynecol Reprod Biol* 76: 117–119.

Bos AF, van Asperen RM, de Leeuw DM, Prechtl HFR. (1997a) The influence of septicaemia on spontaneous motility in preterm infants. *Early Hum Dev* 50: 61–70.

Bos AF, van Loon AJ, Hadders-Algra M, Martijn A, Okken A, Prechtl HFR. (1997b) Spontaneous motility in preterm, small for gestational age infants. II. Qualitative aspects. *Early Hum Dev* 50: 131–147.

Bos AF, van Loon AJ, Martijn A, van Asperen RM, Okken A, Prechtl HFR. (1997c) Spontaneous motility in preterm, small-for-gestational age infants. I. Quantitative aspects. *Early Hum Dev* 50: 115–130.

Bos AF, Martijn A, Okken A, Prechtl HFR. (1998a) Quality of general movements in preterm infants with transient periventricular echodensities. *Acta Paediatr* 87: 328–335.

Bos AF, Martijn A, van Asperen RM, Hadders-Algra M, Okken A, Prechtl HFR. (1998b) Qualitative assessment of general movements in high risk preterm infants with chronic lung disease requiring dexamethasone therapy. *J Pediatr* 132: 300–306.

Bos AF, Einspieler C, Prechtl HFR, Touwen B, Okken-Beukens M, Stremmelar F. (1999) The quality of spontaneous motor activity in preterm infants as early predictive signs for minor neurological abnormalities at two years. *Newsletter Neonat Neurol* 8: 4–5.

Bos AF, Venema IMJ, Bergervoet M, Zweens MJ, Pratl B, van Eykern LA. (2000) Spontaneous motility in preterm infants treated with indomethacin. *Biol Neonat* 78: 174–180.

Bos AF, Einspieler C, Prechtl HFR. (2001) Intrauterine growth retardation, general movements and neurodevelopmental outcome: a review. *Dev Med Child Neurol* 43: 61–68.

Bos AF, Dibiasi J, Tiessen AH, Bergmann KA. (2002a) Treating preterm infants at risk for chronic lung disease with dexamethasone leads to an impaired quality of general movements. *Biol Neonat* 82: 155–158.

Bos AF, Einspieler C, Prechtl HFR. (2002b) Motor repertoire at early age for prediction of neurological deficits at 2 y. *Pediatr Res* 52: 796. (Abstract.)

Bots RSG, Nijhuis JG, Martin CB jr, Prechtl HFR. (1981) Human fetal eye movements: detection in utero by ultrasonography. *Early Hum Dev* 5: 87–94.

Bracci E, Ballerini L, Nistri A. (1996) Spontaneous rhythmic bursts induced by pharmacological block of inhibition in lumbar motoneurons of the neonatal rat spinal cord. *J Neurophysiol* 75: 640–647.

Braddick OJ, Atkinson J. (1983) Some recent findings on the development of human binocularity: a review. *Behav Brain Res* 10: 141–150.

Brandt I. (1983) *Griffiths Entwicklungsskalen (GES) zur Beurteilung der Entwicklung in den ersten beiden Lebensjahren*. Weinheim, Basel: Beltz.

Bregman J, Farrell EE. (1992) Neurodevelopmental outcome in infants with bronchopulmonary dysplasia. *Clin Perinat* 19: 673–694.

Brown LD, Heermann J. (1997) The effect of developmental care on preterm infant outcome. *Appl Nurs Res* 10: 190–197.

Bruininks RH. (1978) *Bruininks Oseretsky Test of Motor Proficiency: Examiner's Manual*. Circle Pines, MN: American Guidance Service.

Brunet O, Lézine I. (1967) *Scala di Sviluppo Psicomotorio della Prima Infanzia*. Firenze: Organizzazioni Special (O.S.)

Buchanan JT. (1982) Identification of interneurons with contralateral, caudal axons in the lamprey spinal cord: synaptic interactions and morphology. *J Neurophysiol* 47: 961–975.

Buchanan JT, Grillner S. (1987) Newly identified 'glutamate interneurons' and their role in locomotion in the lamprey spinal cord. *Science* 236: 312–314.

Cazalets JR, Borde M, Clarac F. (1995) Localization and organization of the central pattern generator for hindlimb locomotion in newborn rat. *J Neurosci* 15: 4943–4951.

Champagnat J, Fortin G. (1997) Primordial respiratory-like rhythm generation in the vertebrate embryo. *TINS* 20: 119–124.

Cheng J, Jovanovic K, Aoyagi Y, Bennett DJ, Han Y, Stein RB. (2002) Differential distribution of interneurons in the neural networks that control walking in the mudpuddy (Nectururs maculaus) spinal cord. *Exp Brain Res* 145: 190–198.

Chugani HT, Phelps ME. (1986) Maturational changes in cerebral function in infants determined by 18FDG positron emission tomography. *Science* 231: 840–843.

Chugani HT, Phelps ME, Mazziotta JC. (1987) 18FDG positron emission tomography in human brain functional development. *Ann Neurol* 22: 487–497.

Cioni G, Prechtl HFR. (1990) Preterm and early postterm motor behaviour in low-risk premature infants. *Early Hum Dev* 23: 159–193.

77

Cioni G, Favilla M, Ghelarducci B, La Noca A. (1984) Development of the dynamic characteristics of the horizontal vestibulo-ocular reflex in infancy. *Neuropediatrics* 15: 125–130.

Cioni G, Ferrari F, Prechtl HFR. (1989) Posture and spontaneous motility in fullterm infants. *Early Hum Dev* 7: 247–262.

Cioni G, Ferrari F, Einspieler C, Paolicelli PB, Barbani MT, Prechtl HFR. (1997a) Comparison between observation of spontaneous movements and neurological examination in preterm infants. *J Pediatr* 130: 704–711.

Cioni G, Paolicelli PB, Rapisardi G, Castellacci AM, Ferrari A. (1997b) Early natural history of spastic diplegia and tetraplegia. *Eur J Pediatr Neurol* 1: 33. (Abstract.)

Cioni G, Prechtl HFR, Ferrari F, Paolicelli PB, Einspieler C, Roversi MF. (1997c) Which better predicts later outcome in fullterm infants: quality of general movements or neurological examination? *Early Hum Dev* 50: 71–85.

Cioni G, Bos AF, Einspieler C, Ferrari F, Martijn A, Paolicelli PB, Rapisardi G, Roversi MF, Prechtl HFR. (2000) Early neurological signs in preterm infants with unilateral intraparenchymal echodensity. *Neuropediatrics* 31: 240–251.

Clyman RI. (1996) Recommendations for the postnatal use of indomethacin: an analysis of four separate treatment strategies. *J Pediatr* 128: 601–607.

Cohen J. (1960) A coefficient of agreement for nominal scales. *Ed Psychol Meas* 20: 37–46.

Coluccini M, Maini S, Sabatini A, Prechtl HFR, Cioni G. (2002) Kinematic analysis of general movements in early infancy. *Dev Med Child Neurol* 44: 14. (Abstract.)

Constantinou JC, Adamson-Macedo EN, Stevenson DK, Mirmiran M, Fleisher BE. (1999) Effects of skin-to-skin holding on general movements of preterm infants. *Clin Pediatr* 38: 467–471.

Cooke RWI, Lucas A, Yudkin PLN, Pryse-Davis J. (1977) Head circumference as an index of brain weight in the fetus and newborn. *Early Hum Dev* 1: 145–149.

Coons S, Guilleminault C. (1985) Motility and arousal in near miss sudden infant death syndrome. *J Pediatr* 107: 728–732.

Cote MP, Gossard JP. (2003) Task-dependent presynaptic inhibition. *J Neurosci* 23: 1886–1893.

Counsell SJ, Allsop JM, Harrison MC, Larkman DJ, Kennea NL, Kapellou O, Cowen FM, Hajnal JV, Edwards AD, Rutherford MA. (2003) Diffusion-weighted imaging of the brain in preterm infants with focal and diffuse white matter abnormality. *Pediatrics* 112: 1–7.

Cummings JJ, D'Eugenio DB, Gross SJ. (1989) A controlled trial of dexamethasone in preterm infants at high risk for bronchopulmonary dysplasia. *NEJM* 320: 1505–1510.

Cunningham JN jr, Carter NW, Rector FZ jr, Seldin DW. (1971) Resting transmembrane potential difference of skeletal muscle in normal subjects and severely ill patients. *J Clin Invest* 50: 49–59.

de Vries JIP, Visser GHA, Prechtl HFR. (1982) The emergence of fetal behaviour. I. Qualitative aspects. *Early Hum Dev* 7: 301–322.

de Vries JIP, Visser GHA, Prechtl HFR. (1984) Fetal motility in the first half of pregnancy. In: Prechtl HFR, editor. *Continuity of Neural Functions from Prenatal to Postnatal Life*. Clin Dev Med 94. Oxford: Blackwell, pp 46–64.

de Vries JIP, Visser GHA, Prechtl HFR. (1985) The emergence of fetal behaviour. II. Quantitative aspects. *Early Hum Dev* 12: 99–120.

de Vries JIP, Visser GHA, Mulder EJH, Prechtl HFR. (1987) Diurnal and other variations in fetal movement and heart rate patterns at 20 to 22 weeks. *Early Hum Dev* 15: 333–348.

de Vries JIP, Visser GHA, Prechtl HFR. (1988) The emergence of fetal behaviour. III. Individual differences and consistencies. *Early Hum Dev* 16: 85–103.

de Vries LS, Regev R, Pennock JM, Wigglesworth JS, Dubowitz LMS. (1988) Ultrasound evolution and later outcome of infants with periventricular densities. *Early Hum Dev* 16: 225–233.

de Vries LS, Dubowitz LMS, Dubowitz V, Pennock JM. (1990) *A Colour Atlas of Brain Disorders in the Newborn*. London: Wolfe.

de Vries LS, Eken P, Dubowitz LMS. (1992) The spectrum of leucomalacia using cranial ultrasound. *Behav Brain Res* 49: 1–6.

de Vries LS, Groenendaal F, Eken P, van Haastert IC, Rademaker KJ, Meiners LC. (1997) Infarcts in the vascular distribution of the middle cerebral artery in preterm and fullterm infants. *Neuropediatrics* 28: 88–96.

Deykin E, Bauman ML, Kelly DH, Hsieh C, Shannon D. (1984) Apnea of infancy and subsequent neurologic, cognitive, and behavioural status. *Pediatrics* 73: 638–645.

Dibiasi J, Einspieler C. (2002) Can spontaneous movements be modulated by visual and acoustic stimulation in 3-month-old infants? *Early Hum Dev* 68: 27–37.

Dibiasi J, Einspieler C. (2004) Load perturbation does not influence spontaneous movements in 3-month-old infants. *Early Hum Dev* 77: 37–46.

DiPietro MA, Broday BA, Teele RL. (1986) Peritrigonal echogenic 'blush' on cranial sonography: pathological correlates. *Am J Roentgenol* 146: 1067–1072.

Doyle LW, Davis PG. (2000) Postnatal corticosteroids in preterm infant: systematic review of effects on mortality and motor function. *J Paediatr Child Health* 36: 101–107.

Dubowitz LMS. (1988) Clinical assessment of infant nervous system. In: Levene MI, Bennett MJ, Punt J, editors. *Fetal and Neonatal Neurology and Neurosurgery*. Edinburgh: Churchill Livingstone, pp 33–40.

Dubowitz LMS, Dubowitz V. (1981) *The Neurological Assessment of the Preterm and Fullterm Newborn Infant*. Clin Dev Med 79. London: Heinemann.

Dubowitz L, Dubowitz V, Palmer P, Miller G, Fawer C, Levene M. (1984) Correlation of neurological assessment in the premature newborn infant with outcome at 1 year. *J Pediatr* 105: 452–456.

Dubowitz LMS, Dubowitz V, Mercuri E. (1999) *The Neurological Assessment of the Preterm and Full-Term Newborn Infant*, 2nd edition. Clin Dev Med 148. Cambridge: Cambridge University Press.

Einspieler C. (1994) Abnormal spontaneous movements in infants with repeated sleep apnoeas. *Early Hum Dev* 36: 31–48.

Einspieler C. (1995) Are repeated sleep apnoeas harmful to the infant's brain? In: Rognum TO, editor. *Sudden Infant Death Syndrome: New Trends in the Nineties*. Oslo: Scandinavian University Press, pp 226–229.

Einspieler C, Prechtl HFR, van Eykern L, de Roos B. (1994) Observation of movements during sleep in ALTE and apnoeic infants. *Early Hum Dev* 40: 39–50.

Einspieler C, Prechtl HFR, Ferrari F, Cioni G, Bos AF. (1997) The qualitative assessment of general movements in preterm, term and young infants – review of the methodology. *Early Hum Dev* 50: 47–60.

Einspieler C, Cioni G, Paolicelli PB, Bos AF, Dressler A, Ferrari F, Roversi MF, Prechtl HFR. (2002) The early markers for later dyskinetic cerebral palsy are different from those for spastic cerebral palsy. *Neuropediatrics* 33: 73–78.

Einspieler C, Kerr AM, Prechtl HFR. (2004) Is the early development of girls with Rett disorder really normal? *Ped Res*.

Eken P, Toet MC, Groenedaal F, de Vries LS. (1995) Predictive value of early neuroimaging, pulsed Doppler, and neurophysiology in fullterm infants with hypoxic-ischaemic encephalopathy. *Arch Dis Child* 73: F75–F80.

Erkinjuntti M. (1988) Body movements during sleep in healthy and neurologically damaged infants. *Early Hum Dev* 16: 283–292.

Estan J, Hope P. (1997) Unilateral neonatal cerebral infarction in fullterm infants. *Arch Dis Child* 76: F88–F93.

Farrell PA, Weiner GM, Lemons JA. (2002) SIDS, ALTE, apnea, and the use of home monitors. *Pediatr Rev* 23: 3–9.

Fazzi E, Orcesi S, Caffi L, Ometto A, Rondini G, Telesca C, Lanzi G. (1994) Neurodevelopmental outcome at 5–7 years in preterm infants with periventricular leukomalacia. *Neuropediatrics* 25: 134–139.

Ferrari F, Cioni,C, Prechtl HFR. (1990) Qualitative changes of general movements in preterm infants with brain lesions. *Early Hum Dev* 23: 193–233.

Ferrari F, Prechtl HFR, Cioni G, Roversi MF, Einspieler C, Gallo C, Paolicelli PB, Cavazutti GB. (1997) Behavioural states, posture and spontaneous movements in infants affected by brain malformation. *Early Hum Dev* 50: 87–113.

Ferrari F, Cioni G, Einspieler C, Roversi MF, Bos AF, Paolocelli PB, Ranzi A, Prechtl HFR. (2002) Cramped synchronised general movements in preterm infants as an early marker for cerebral palsy. *Arch Pediatr Adolesc Med* 156: 460–467.

Fok M, Stein RB. (2002) Effects of cholinergic and noradrenergic agents on locomotion in the mudpuppy (Necturus maculates). *Exp Brain Res* 145: 498–504.

Forssberg H. (1999) Neural control of human motor development. *Curr Opin Neurobiol* 9: 676–682.

Geerdink JJ, Hopkins B. (1993a) Qualitative changes in general movements and their prognostic values in preterm infants. *Eur J Paediatr* 152: 362–367.

Geerdink JJ, Hopkins B. (1993b) Effects of birth weight status and gestational age on the quality of general movements in preterm newborns. *Biol Neonat* 63: 215–224.

Gesell A. (1945) *Embryology of Behavior*. New York: Harper and Brothers. (Reprinted 1988. Cambridge: Cambridge University Press.)

Graham-Brown T. (1913) On the nature of fundamental activity of the nervous centre; together with an analysis of the conditioning of rhythmic activity in progression, and a theory of the evolution of function in the nervous system. *J Physiol* 47: 18–45.

Gray C, Davies F, Molyneux E. (1999) Apparent life-threatening events presenting to a pediatric emergency department. *Pediatr Emerg Care* 15: 195–199.

Griffiths R. (1954) *The Ability of Babies*. London: London University Press.

Grillner S. (1999) Bridging the gap – from ion channels to networks and behaviour. *Curr Opin Neurobiol* 9: 663–669.

Guzzetta A, Mercuri E, Rapisardi G, Ferrari F, Roversi F, Cowan F, Rutherford M, Paolicelli PB, Einspieler C, Boldrini A, Dubowitz L, Prechtl HFR, Cioni G. (2003) General movements detect early signs of hemiplegia in term infants with neonatal cerebral infarction. *Neuropediatrics* 34: 61–66.

Hadders-Algra M. (1993) General movements in early infancy: what do they tell us about the nervous system? *Early Hum Dev* 34: 29–37.

Hadders-Algra M, Groothuis AM. (1999) Quality of general movements in infancy is related to neurological dysfunction, ADHD, and aggressive behaviour. *Dev Med Child Neurol* 41: 381–391.

Hadders-Algra M, Prechtl HFR. (1992) Developmental course of general movements in early infancy. I. Descriptive analysis of change in form. *Early Hum Dev* 28: 201–213.

Hadders-Algra M, Prechtl HFR. (1993) EMG correlates of general movements in healthy preterm infants. *J Physiol* 459: 330. (Abstract.)

Hadders-Algra M, Huisjes HJ, Touwen BCL. (1988) Preterm or small-for-gestational-age infants. Neurological and behavioural development at the age of 6 years. *Eur J Pediatr* 147: 460–467.

Hadders-Algra M, van Eykern LA, Klip-van den Nieuwendijk AW, Prechtl HFR. (1992) Developmental course of general movements in early infancy. II. EMG correlates. *Early Hum Dev* 28: 231–251.

Hadders-Algra M, Nakae Y, van Eykern LA, Klip-van den Nieuwendijk AW, Prechtl HFR. (1993) The effect of behavioural state on general movements in healthy term newborns. A polymyographic study. *Early Hum Dev* 35: 63–79.

Hadders-Algra M, Bos AF, Martijn A, Prechtl HFR. (1994) Infantile chorea in an infant with severe bronchopulmonary dysplasia: an EMG study. *Dev Med Child Neurol* 36: 177–182.

Hadders-Algra M, Klip-van den Nieuwendijk AW, Martijn A, van Eykern LA. (1997) Assessment of general movements: towards a better understanding of a sensitive method to evaluate brain function in young infants. *Dev Med Child Neurol* 39: 88–98.

Hagberg B, Hagberg G. (1993) The origins of cerebral palsy. In: David TJ, editor. *Recent Advances in Paediatrics*. Edinburgh and London: Churchill Livingstone, pp 67–83.

Hagberg B, Aicardi J, Dias K, Ramos O. (1983) A progressive syndrome of autism, dementia, ataxia, and loss of purposeful hand use in girls: Rett's syndrome: report on 35 cases. *Ann Neurol* 14: 471–479.

Hagberg B, Hagberg G, Olow I, van Wendt L. (1996) The changing panorama of cerebral palsy in Sweden. VII. Prevalence and origin in the birth year period 1987–90. *Acta Paediatr* 85: 954–960.

Hasselgren PO, Pedersen P, Sax HC, Warner BW, Fischer JE. (1988) Current concepts of protein turnover and amino acid transport in liver and skeletal muscle during sepsis. *Arch Surg* 123: 992–999.

Hines RB, Minde K, Marton P. (1980) Behavioral development of premature infants: an ethological approach. *Dev Med Child Neurol* 22: 623–632.

Hooker D. (1952) *The Prenatal Origin of Behavior*. Lawrence: University of Kansas Press.

Hopkins B, Prechtl HFR. (1984) A qualitative approach to the development of movements during early infancy. In: Prechtl HFR, editor. *Continuity of Neural Functions from Prenatal to Postnatal Life*. Clin Dev Med 94. Oxford: Blackwell, pp 179–197.

Illingworth RS. (1966) The diagnosis of cerebral palsy in the first year of life. *Dev Med Child Neurol* 8: 178–194.

Irwin CO. (1932) The amount of motility of 73 newborn infants. *J Comp Psychol* 14: 415–428.

Iwayama K, Eishima M. (1997) Neonatal sucking behavior and its development until 14 months. *Early Hum Dev* 47: 1–9.

Jovanovic L, Druzin M, Peterson CM. (1981) Effect of euglycemia on the outcome of pregnancy in insulin-dependent diabetic women as compared with normal control subjects. *Am J Med* 71: 921–930.

Kahn A, Dan B, Groswasser J, Franco P, Sottiaux M. (1996) Normal sleep architecture in infants and children. *J Clin Neurophysiol* 13: 184–197.

Kainer F, Prechtl HFR, Engele H, Einspieler C. (1997) Prenatal and postnatal assessment of the quality of general movements in infants of women with type-I diabetes mellitus. *Early Hum Dev* 50: 13–25.

Kakebeeke TH, von Siebenthal K, Largo RH. (1997) Differences in movement quality at term among preterm and term infants. *Biol Neonat* 71: 367–378.

Kakebeeke TH, von Siebenthal K, Largo RH. (1998) Movement quality in preterm infants prior to term. *Biol Neonat* 73: 145–154.

Kerr AM. (1995) Early clinical signs in Rett disorder. *Neuropediatrics* 26: 67–71.

Largo RH. (1993) *Babyjahre. Die frühkindliche Entwicklung aus biologischer Sicht.* Hamburg: Carlsen.

Largo RH, Graf S, Kundu S, Hunziker U, Molinari L. (1990) Predicting developmental outcome at school age from infant tests of normal, at-risk and retarded infants. *Dev Med Child Neurol* 32: 30–45.

Laurini RN, Visser GH, van Ballegooie E. (1984) Morphological fetoplacental abnormalities despite well-controlled diabetic pregnancy. *Lancet* 7: 800. (Letter.)

Levene MI. (1990) Cerebral ultrasound and neurological impairment: telling the future. *Arch Dis Child* 65: 469–471.

Levene MI, Fawer CL, Lamont RF. (1982) Risk factors in the development of intraventricular haemorrhage in the preterm neonate. *Arch Dis Child* 57: 410–417.

Leviton A, Paneth N. (1990) White matter damage in preterm newborns – an epidemiologic perspective. *Early Hum Dev* 24: 1–22.

Lorenz K. (1971) Gestalt perception as a source of scientific knowledge. (English translation from a German paper in 1959.) In: Lorenz K, editor. *Studies in Animal and Human Behaviour.* Vol II. London: Methuen, pp 281–322.

Löscher WN, Einspieler C, Klug EM, Haidmayer R, Gallasch E, Kurz R, Kenner T. (1990) Neurological status, sleep apnoea frequency and blood oxygenation in 6-week-old infants. *Early Hum Dev* 24: 119–130.

MacFarlane CM, Tsakalakos N. (1985) Evidence of hyperinsulinaemia and hypoxaemia in the cord blood of neonates born to mothers with gestational diabetes. *S Afr Med J* 67: 81–84.

McGraw MB. (1943) *The Neuromuscular Maturation of the Human Infant.* New York: Columbia University Press.

Ment LR, Oh W, Ehrenkranz RA, Philip AGS, Vohr B, Allan W, Duncan CC, Scott DT, Taylor KJW, Katz KH, Schneider KC, Makuch RW. (1994) Low-dose indomethacin and prevention of intraventricular haemorrhage: a multicenter randomized trial. *Pediatrics* 93: 543–550.

Mercuri E, Dubowitz L. (1996) The prognosis of neonatal neurological abnormalities. *Baillieres Clin Paediatr* 4: 394–409.

Metz CE. (1978) Basic principles of ROC analysis. *Semin Nucl Med* 8: 283–298.

Minkowski M. (1928) Neurobiologische Studien am menschlichen Fötus. *Handbuch der biologischen Arbeitsmethoden* 5: 511–618.

Mizrahi EM, Kellaway P. (1987) Characterization and classification of neonatal seizures. *Neurology* 37: 1837–1884.

Mizrahi EM, Kellaway P. (1998) *Diagnosis and Management of Neonatal Seizures.* Philadelphia: Lippincott Raven.

Molteno C, Grosz P, Wallace P, Jones M. (1995) Neurological examination of the preterm and full-term infant at risk for developmental disabilities using the Dubowitz neurological assessment. *Early Hum Dev* 41: 167–176.

Mulder EJH. (1992) Diabetic pregnancy. In: Nijhuis JG, editor. Fetal Behaviour: *Development and Perinatal Aspects.* Oxford: Medical Publications, pp 193–200.

Naidu S, Hyman S, Harris EL. Narayanan V, Johns D, Castora F. (1995) Rett syndrome studies of natural history and search for a genetic marker. *Neuropediatrics* 26: 63–66.

Navarrete R, Slawinska U, Vrbova G. (2002) Electromyographic activity patterns of ankle flexor and extensor muscles during spontaneous and L-DOPA-induced locomotion in freely moving neonatal rats. *Exp Neurol* 173: 256–265.

Nelson CA, Wewerka S, Thomas KM, Tribby-Walbridge S, deRegnier R, Georgieff M. (2000) Neurocognitive sequelae of infants of diabetic mothers. *Behav Neurosci* 114: 950–956.

Nijhuis JG, Prechtl HFR, Martin CB jr, Bots RSGM. (1982) Are there behavioural states in the human fetus? *Early Hum Dev* 6: 177–195.

Nishimaru H, Izuka M, Ozaki S, Kudo N. (1996) Spontaneous motoneuronal activity mediated by glycine and GABA in the spinal cord of rat fetuses in vitro. *J Physiol* 497: 131–143.

Okado N, Kojima T. (1984) Ontogeny of the central nervous system: neurogenesis, fibre connection, synaptogenesis and myelination in the spinal cord. In: Prechtl HFR, editor. *Continuity of Neural Functions from Prenatal to Postnatal Life.* Clin Dev Med 94. Oxford: Blackwell, pp 31–46.

Onimaru H. (1995) Studies of the respiratory center using isolated brainstem-spinal cord preparations. *Neurosci Res* 21: 183–190.

Oppenheim RW (1984) Ontogenetic adaptations in neural and behavioural development, towards a more 'ecological' developmental psychobiology. In: Prechtl HFR, editor. *Continuity of Neural Functions from Prenatal to Postnatal Life*. Clin Dev Med 94. Oxford: Blackwell, pp 16–30.

Ornoy A, Cohen E. (1996) Outcome of children born to epileptic mothers treated with carbamazepine during pregnancy. *Arch Dis Child* 75: 517–520.

Palisano R, Rosenbaum P, Walter S, Russel S, Wood E, Galuppi B. (1997) Development and reliability of a system to classify gross motor function in children with cerebral palsy. *Dev Med Child Neurol* 39: 214–223.

Parisi P, Francia A, Vanacore N, Fiore S, Giallonardo AT, Manfredi M. (2003) Psychomotor development and general movements in offspring of women with epilepsy and anticonvulsant therapy. *Early Hum Dev* 74: 97–108.

Penney GC, Mair G, Pearson DW; Scottish Diabetes in Pregnancy Group. (2003) Outcomes of pregnancies in women with type 1 diabetes in Scotland: a national population-based study. *Br J Obstet Gynaecol* 110: 315–318.

Percy AK. (1995) Rett syndrome. *Curr Opin Neurol* 8: 156–160.

Perlman JM. (1998) White matter injury in the preterm infant: an important determination of abnormal neurodevelopmental outcome. *Early Hum Dev* 53: 99–120.

Persson B, Hanson U. (1996) Fetal size at birth in relation to quality of blood glucose control in pregnancies complicated by pregestational diabetes mellitus. *Br J Obstet Gynaecol* 103: 427–433.

Petry CD, Wobken JD, McKay H, Eaton MA, Seybold VS, Johnson DE, Georgieff MK. (1994) Placental transferrin receptor in diabetic pregnancies with increased fetal iron demand. *Am J Physiol* 267: E507–E514.

Prechtl HFR. (1958) The directed head turning response and allied movements of the human body. *Behavior* 8: 212–242.

Prechtl HFR. (1974) The behavioural state of the newborn (a review). Duivenvoorde Lecture. *Brain Res* 76: 185–212.

Prechtl HFR. (1977) *The Neurological Examination of the Full-term Newborn Infant*, 2nd edition. Clin Dev Med 63. London: Heinemann.

Prechtl HFR. (1980) The optimality concept. *Early Hum Dev* 4: 201–205.

Prechtl HFR. (1984a) *Continuity of Neural Functions from Prenatal to Postnatal Life*. Clin Dev Med 94. Oxford: Blackwell.

Prechtl HFR. (1984b) Continuity and change in early neural development. In: Prechtl HFR, editor. *Continuity of Neural Functions from Prenatal to Postnatal Life*. Clin Dev Med 94. Oxford: Blackwell, pp 1–15.

Prechtl HFR. (1986) New perspectives in early human development. *Eur J Obstet Gynecol Reprod Biol* 21: 347–355.

Prechtl HFR. (1989a) Development of postural control in infancy. In: von Euler C, Forssberg H, Lagercrantz H, editors. *Neurobiology of Early Infant Behaviour*. Wenner-Gren Intern Symp Series Vol 55. London: Macmillan, pp 59–68.

Prechtl HFR. (1989b) Fetal behaviour. In: Hill A, Volpe J, editors. *Fetal Neurology*. New York: Raven Press, pp 1–16.

Prechtl HFR. (1990) Qualitative changes of spontaneous movements in fetus and preterm infant are a marker of neurological dysfunction. *Early Hum Dev* 23: 151–158.

Prechtl HFR. (1992) Some remarks on the neonate. In: Nijhuis JG, editor. *Fetal Behaviour: Developmental and Perinatal Aspects*. Oxford: Medical Publications, pp 65–72.

Prechtl HFR. (1997a) State of the art of a new functional assessment of the young nervous system. An early predictor of cerebral palsy. *Early Hum Dev* 50: 1–11.

Prechtl HFR. (1997b) The importance of fetal movements. In: Connolly KJ, Forssberg H, editors. *Neurophysiology and Psychology of Motor Development*. Clin Dev Med 143/144. Cambridge: Cambridge University Press, pp 42–53.

Prechtl HFR. (1999) How can we assess the integrity of the fetal nervous system? In: Arbeille P, Manlik D, Laurini RN, editors. *Fetal Hypoxia*. New York and London: Parthenon, pp 109–115.

Prechtl HFR. (2001a) General movement assessment as a method of developmental neurology: new paradigms and their consequences. The 1999 Ronnie MacKeith Lecture. *Dev Med Child Neurol* 43: 836–842.

Prechtl HFR. (2001b) Prenatal and early postnatal development of human motor behaviour. In: Kalverboer

AF, Gramsbergen A, editors. *Handbook of Brain and Behaviour in Human Development.* Amsterdam: Kluwer, pp 415–427.

Prechtl HFR, Beintema DJ. (1964) *The Neurological Examination of the Fullterm Newborn Infant.* London: Heinemann.

Prechtl HFR, Einspieler C. (1997) Is neurological assessment of the fetus possible? *Eur J Obstet Gynecol Repr Biol* 75: 81–84.

Prechtl HFR, Hopkins B. (1986) Developmental transformations of spontaneous movements in early infancy. *Early Hum Dev* 14: 233–238.

Prechtl HFR, Lenard HG. (1968) Verhaltensphysiologie des Neugeborenen. In: Linneweh F, editor. *Fortschritte der Pädologie.* Vol II. Berlin: Springer, pp 88–122.

Prechtl HFR, Nolte R (1984) Motor behaviour of preterm infants. In: Prechtl HFR, editor. *Continuity of Neural Functions from Prenatal to Postnatal Life.* Clin Dev Med 94. Oxford: Blackwell, pp 79–92.

Prechtl HFR, Fargel JW, Weinmann HM, Bakker HH. (1979) Postures, motility and respiration of low-risk preterm infants. *Dev Med Child Neurol* 21: 3–27.

Prechtl HFR, Ferrari F, Cioni G. (1993) Predictive value of general movements in asphyxiated fullterm infants. *Early Hum Dev* 35: 91–120.

Prechtl HFR, Bos AF, Cioni G, Einspieler C, Ferrari F. (1997a) *Spontaneous Motor Activity as a Diagnostic Tool.* Demonstration Video. London and Graz: The GM Trust.

Prechtl HFR, Einspieler C, Cioni G, Bos AF, Ferrari F, Sontheimer D. (1997b) An early marker for neurological deficits after perinatal brain lesions. *Lancet* 349: 1361–1363.

Prechtl HFR, Cioni G, Einspieler C, Bos AF, Ferrari F. (2001) Role of vision on early motor development: lessons from the blind. *Dev Med Child Neurol* 43: 198–201.

Preyer W. (1885) *Die spezielle Physiologie des Embryo.* Leipzig: Grieben.

Rademaker KJ, Groenendaal F, Jansen GH, Ekken P, de Vries LS. (1994) Unilateral haemorrhagic parenchymal lesions in the preterm infant: shape, site, and prognosis. *Acta Paediatr* 83: 602–608.

Rapisardi G, Cappellini M, Luce Cioni M, Ernst C, Fonda C. (2002) Prognostic value of combined use of general movement assessment and proton magnetic resonance spectroscopy in term infants affected by hypoxic-ischemic encephalopathy. *Brain Dev* 24: 395. (Abstract.)

Reuwer PJH, Sijmons EA, Rietman GW, van Tiel MWM, Bruinse HW. (1987) Intrauterine growth retardation: prediction of perinatal distress by Doppler ultrasound. *Lancet* 22: 415–418.

Ribbert LSM, Visser GHA, Mulder EJH, Zonneveld MF, Morssink LP. (1993) Changes with time in fetal heart rate variation, movement incidences and haemodynamics in intrauterine growth retarded fetuses: a longitudinal approach to the assessment of fetal well being. *Early Hum Dev* 31: 195–208.

Rizzo T, Ogata ES, Dooley SL, Metzger BE, Cho NH. (1994) Perinatal complications and cognitive development in two- to five-year-old children of diabetic mothers. *Am J Obstet Gynecol* 171: 706–713.

Roberts A, Perrins R. (1995) Positive feedback as a general mechanism for sustaining rhythmic and non-rhythmic activity. *J Physiol* 89: 241–248.

Roodenburg PJ, Wladimiroff JW, van Es A, Prechtl HFR. (1991) Classification and quantitative aspects of fetal movements during the second half of normal pregnancy. *Early Hum Dev* 25: 19–35.

Sackett DL, Straus SE, Richardson WS, Rosenberg W, Haynes RB. (2000) *Evidence-Based Medicine. How Do You Practice and Teach EBM,* 2nd edition. Edinburgh: Churchill Livingstone, pp 67–93.

Sadreyev RI, Panchin YV. (2002) Effects of glutamate agonists on the isolated neurons from the locomotor network of the mollusc Clione limacine. *Neuroreport* 13: 2235–2239.

Sarnat HB, Sarnat MS. (1976) Neonatal encephalopathy following fetal distress. A clinical and electroencephalographic study. *Arch Neurol* 33: 696–705.

Schechtman VL, Harper RM, Wilson AJ, Southall DP. (1992) Sleep state organization in normal infants and victims of the sudden infant death syndrome. *Pediatrics* 89: 865–870.

Scolnik D, Nulman I, Rovet J, Gladstone D, Czuchta D, Gardner HA, Gladstone R, Ashby P, Weksberg R, Einarson T. (1994) Neurodevelopment of children exposed in utero to phenytoin and carbamazepine monotherapy. *JAMA* 271: 767–770.

Sherrington C. (1906) *The Integrative Action of the Central Nervous System.* New York: Scribners. (Reprinted 1961. New Haven: Yale University Press.)

Shinwell ES, Karplus M, Reich D, Weintraub Z, Blazer S, Bader D, Yurman S, Dolfin T, Kogan A, Dollberg S, Arbel E, Goldberg M, Gur I, Naor N, Sirota L, Mogilner S, Zaritsky A, Barak M, Gottfried E. (2000) Early postnatal dexamethasone treatment and increased incidence of cerebral palsy. *Arch Dis Child* 83: F177–F181.

Shiono S, Fantini GA, Roberts JP, Chiao J, Shires GT. (1989) Assessment of the early cellular membrane response to live Escherichia coli bacteraemia. *J Surg Res* 46: 9–15.

Sival DA, Visser GHA, Prechtl HFR. (1992a) The effect of intrauterine growth retardation on the quality of general movements in the human fetus. *Early Hum Dev* 28: 119–132.

Sival DA, Visser GHA, Prechtl HFR. (1992b) The relationship between the quantity and quality of prenatal movements in pregnancies complicated by intrauterine growth retardation and premature rupture of the membranes. *Early Hum Dev* 30: 193–209.

Sival DA, Brouwer OF, Meiners LC, Sauer PJJ, Prechtl HFR, Bos AF. (2003) The influence of cerebral malformations on the quality of general movements in spina bifida aperta. *Eur J Pediatr Surg* 13: S29–S30.

Spitzer NC. (1995) Spontaneous activity: functions of calcium transients in neuronal differentiation. *Perspect Dev Neurobiol* 2: 379–386.

Staras K, Kemenes I, Benjamin PR, Kemenes G. (2003) Loss of self-inhibition is a cellular mechanism for episodic rhythmic behaviour. *Curr Biol* 13: 116–124.

Stevens B, Petryshen P, Hawkins J, Smith B, Taylor P. (1996) Developmental versus conventional care: a comparison of clinical outcomes for very low birth weight infants. *Can J Nurs Res* 28: 97–113.

Suster ML, Bate M. (2002) Embryonic assembly of a central pattern generator without sensory input. *Nature* 416: 174–178.

Suzue T. (1984) Respiratory rhythm generation in the vitro brain stem – spinal cord preparation of the neonatal rat. *J Physiol* 354: 173–183.

Taft LT. (1995) Cerebral palsy. *Pediatr Rev* 16: 411–418.

Takahashi M, Alford S. (2002) The requirement of presynaptic metabotropic glutamate receptors for the maintenance of locomotion. *J Neurosci* 22: 3692–3999.

Teberg AJ, Walther FJ, Pena IC. (1988) Mortality, morbidity, and outcome of the small-for-gestational age infant. *Semin Perinatol* 12: 84–94.

Thomas A, Saint-Anne Dargassies S. (1952) *Etudes Neurologiques sur le Nouveau-né et le Jeune Nourisson.* Paris: Masson.

Topp M, Langhoff-Roos J, Uldall P, Kristensen J. (1996) Intrauterine growth and gestational age in preterm infants with cerebral palsy. *Early Hum Dev* 44: 27–36.

Touwen BCL. (1976) *Neurological Development in Infancy.* Clin Dev Med 58. London: Heinemann.

Touwen BCL. (1979) *Examination of the Child with Minor Neurological Dysfunction*, 2nd edition. Clin Dev Med 71. London: Heinemann.

Touwen BCL. (1990) Variability and stereotypy of spontaneous motility as a predictor of neurological development of preterm infants. *Dev Med Child Neurol* 32: 501–509.

Trevarthen E, Moser HW. (1988) Diagnostic criteria for Rett syndrome. *Ann Neurol* 23: 425–428.

Tsubokura H. (2002) Clinical significance of general movements. *No To Hattatsu* 34: 122–128.

Tsubota S, Adachi N, Chen JF, Yorozuya T, Nagaro T, Arai T. (1999) Dexamethasone changes brain monoamine metabolism and aggravates ischemic neuronal damage in rats. *Anesthesiol* 90: 515–523.

Tuor UI, Simone CS, Barks JD, Post M. (1993) Dexamethasone prevents cerebral infarction without affecting cerebral blood flow in neonatal rats. *Stroke* 24: 452–457.

Uvebrant P, Hagberg G. (1992) Intrauterine growth in children with cerebral palsy. *Acta Paediatr* 81: 407–412.

van der Heide JC, Paolicelli PB, Boldrini A, Cioni G. (1999) Kinematic and qualitative analysis of lower-extremity movements in preterm infants with brain lesions. *Phys Ther* 79: 546–557.

van Kranen-Mastenbroek V, van Oostenbrugge R, Palmans L, Stevens A, Kingma H, Blanco C, Hasaart T, Vles J. (1992) Inter- and intra-observer agreement in the assessment of the quality of spontaneous movements in the newborn. *Brain Dev* 14: 289–293.

van Kranen-Mastenbroek V, Kingma H, Caberg H, Ghys A, Blanco CE, Hasaart THM, Vles JSH. (1994) Quality of spontaneous general movements in full-term small for gestational age and appropriate for gestational age newborn infants. *Neuropediatrics* 25: 145–153.

van Wulfften Palthe T, Hopkins B. (1984) Development of the infant's social competence during early face-to-face interaction: a longitudinal study. In: Prechtl HFR, editor. *Continuity of Neural Functions from Prenatal to Postnatal Life.* Clin Dev Med 94. Oxford: Blackwell, pp 198–219.

Vining EPG, Accardo PJ, Rubenstein JE, Farrell SE, Roizen NJ. (1976) Cerebral palsy. A pediatric developmentalist's overview. *Am J Dis Child* 130: 643–649.

Visser GHA, Laurini RN, de Vries JIP, Prechtl HFR. (1985) Abnormal motor behaviour in anencephalic fetuses. *Early Hum Dev* 11: 221–229.

Volpe JJ. (1989) Intraventricular haemorrhage in the premature infant – current concepts. Part II. *Ann Neurol* 25: 109–116.

Volpe JJ. (1995) *Neurology of the Newborn*, 3rd edition. Philadelphia: WB Saunders Company.

Volpe JJ. (2000) *Neurology of the Newborn*, 4th edition. Philadelphia: WB Saunders Company.

von Bernuth H, Prechtl HFR. (1969) Vestibular-ocular response and its state dependency in newborn infants. *Neuropädiatrie* 1: 11–24.

von Holst E. (1939) Die relative Koordination als Phänomen und Methode zentralnervöser Funktionsanalyse. In: Asher L, Spiro K, editors. *Ergebnisse der Physiologie*. München: Bergmann, pp 228–306.

Walther FJ. (1988) Growth and development of term disproportionate small-for-gestational age infants at the age of 7 years. *Early Hum Dev* 18: 1–11.

Westfall MV, Sayeed MM. (1988) Basal and insulin-stimulated skeletal muscle sugar transport in endotoxic and bacteremic rats. *Am J Physiol* 254: R673–R679.

Witt-Engerström I. (1987) Rett syndrome: a retrospective pilot study on potential early predictive symptomatology. *Brain Dev* 9: 481–486.

Wulfeck BB, Trauner DA, Tallal PA. (1991) Neurological, cognitive and linguistic features of infants after early stroke. *Pediatr Neurol* 7: 266–269.

Yuge M, Okano S, Tachibana K, Hojo M, Kawamoto M, Suzuki J. (2001) Assessment of general movement at routine medical examination of one-month-old infants. *No To Hattatsu* 33: 246–252.

Zubrick SR, Kurinczuk JJ, McDermott BMC, McKelvey RS, Silburn SR, Davies LS. (2000) Fetal growth and subsequent mental health problems in children aged 4 to 13 years. *Dev Med Child Neurol* 42: 14–20.

INDEX